21-DAY Tummy DIET COOKBOOK

150 All-New Recipes That Shrink, Soothe, and Satisfy

BY LIZ VACCARIELLO

WITH **KATE SCARLATA, RD**

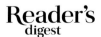

The Reader's Digest Association, Inc.
New York, NY/Montreal

A READER'S DIGEST BOOK
Copyright © 2013 The Reader's Digest Association, Inc.
All rights reserved. Unauthorized reproduction, in any manner, is prohibited.
Reader's Digest is a registered trademark of The Reader's Digest Association, Inc.

Food photographs by Andrew Purcell
Food styling by Carrie Purcell
Prop styling and chalk art by Sarah Cave
Test team photographs by Steve Vaccariello

Library of Congress Cataloging-in-Publication Data
Vaccariello, Liz.
  21-day tummy diet cookbook : 150 all-new recipes that shrink, soothe and satisfy / by Liz
Vaccariello with Kate Scarlata, RD.
     pages cm -- (N/a)
  title: Twenty-one-day tummy diet cookbook
  Summary: "Belly bulges plague millions of Americans. So does bloating, heartburn, and other
tummy troubles. In 21-Day Tummy Diet Cookbook. there are 150 all-new quick and easy recipes
to help you extend and maintain the 21-Day Tummy Diet. Featuring sample menus for each
phase, easy to follow tips on how to create your own Belly Buddy recipes, and inspirational
stories from the Tummy Testers, who collectively lost 90 pounds in 3 weeks, shed 29 inches
from their waists, and reported fewer digestive symptoms and happier tummies"-- Provided by
publisher.
  ISBN 978-1-62145-139-6 (hardback)
1. Reducing diets--Recipes. 2. Weight loss. 3. Abdomen. I. Scarlata, Kate. II. Reader's Digest
Association. III. Title. IV. Title: Twenty-one-day tummy diet cookbook.
  RM222.2.V245 2014
  641.5'638--dc23
                          2014026970

We are committed to both the quality of our products and the service we provide to our
customers. We value your comments, so please feel free to contact us.

     The Reader's Digest Association, Inc.
     Adult Trade Publishing
     44 South Broadway
     White Plains, NY 10601

For more Reader's Digest products and information, visit our website:
     www.rd.com (in the United States)
     www.readersdigest.ca (in Canada)

Printed in China

3 5 7 9 10 8 6 4 2

NOTE TO OUR READERS
The information in this book should not be substituted for, or used to alter, medical therapy
without your doctor's advice. For a specific health problem, consult your physician for guidance.

Contents

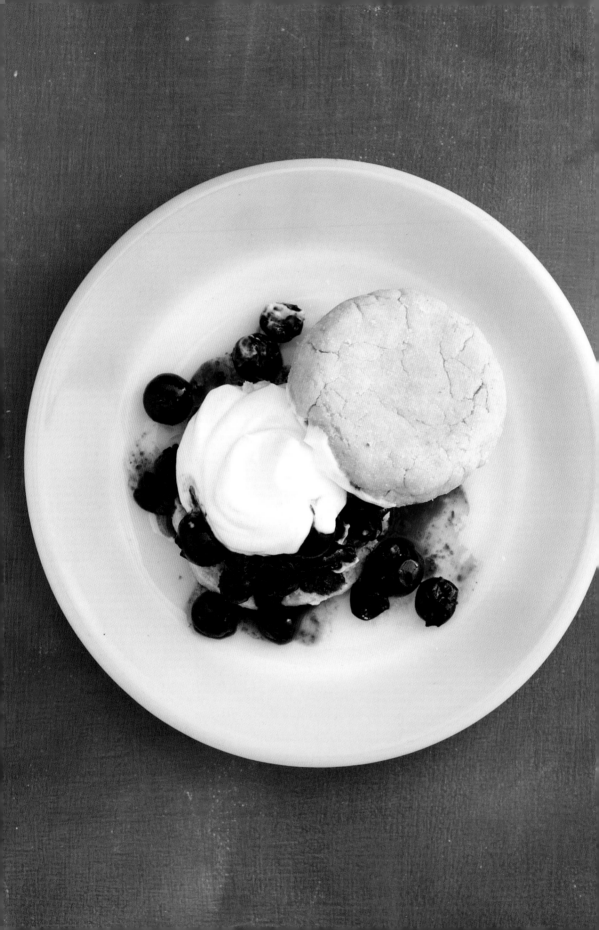

Introduction

I'm fortunate to have had a lot of blessings in my life—a devoted husband, healthy and happy children, and a job I adore. As editor in chief of *Reader's Digest*, I get a front-row seat to the front lines of what's happening in America and around the world. I get to hear from folks like you about your concerns and your interests, and I have the privilege of finding and delivering information you can use to live your best lives. That is what Reader's Digest magazine and books have been doing for more than 90 years.

With my background as a health journalist, I knew that losing weight, especially stubborn belly fat, was a daily struggle for many of you. But it wasn't until recently that I realized how closely these weight issues were related to other stomach problems—the belly grumbles of digestive discord—and just how many of you have been suffering, all too often in silence. So I went looking for a solution.

I uncovered a connection that scientists are just beginning to understand: The bacteria in your gut play a huge role in inflammation, tummy fat, and digestive woes. Moreover, what you eat can directly affect both your gut flora and the inflammatory response in your cells. This is the latest in cutting-edge medical science—you can say you heard it here first!

To combine this revolutionary science with real-life eating, I enlisted Kate Scarlata, a registered dietitian with 25 years of experience in treating digestive health. After extensive intestinal surgery, Kate experienced firsthand the aftermath of gut bacteria imbalance, which made her belly bloated and crampy. So she has a personal interest in keeping up with the latest digestive health research. She has helped countless clients (and herself) get a grip on their tummy troubles and, with the *21-Day Tummy Diet Cookbook*, she will help you, too.

Since many of the same foods that trigger gastrointestinal (GI) symptoms also create belly fat, the revolutionary 21-Day

Tummy plan was carefully designed to eliminate them. But it doesn't stop there. The plan also puts an emphasis on consuming key nutritious foods that ease digestive woes and make weight loss easier. That's right, finally a diet that combats common GI problems and weight gain *at the same time!*

The 21-Day Tummy plan works. How do we know? I tried it myself and recruited 11 other testers, and our results were outstanding! Yes, we flattened our bellies; yes, we calmed our digestive systems; and yes, we whittled away the inches. The grand total of weight loss by our test team in 3 weeks was a whopping 90 pounds! One of our testers, Rob McMahon, lost 19 pounds, almost a pound a day, in just 21 days.

Did we lose belly inches? You bet. The test team lost a grand total of 29 inches off their waistlines. One panelist, Gregg Roth, lost 4½ inches off his midsection. Talk about moving his belt notch! Dorothy Nuzzo, another tester, trimmed 2¼ inches from her waist and dropped four dress sizes! I lost 10 inches overall and 10 pounds. I am sure you will be successful, too.

What was truly remarkable was the disappearance of nagging digestive symptoms. In fact, every single one of us reported improved digestion. We saw a reduction in heartburn, pain, gas, bloating, constipation, and diarrhea—and believe me, we were more than happy to say good-bye to those troubling digestive issues. In fact, two of our testers, Rob McMahon and Phyllis Gebhardt, discontinued using daily acid reflux medications.

I have never really had a weight problem, and my digestion has always treated me pretty well. But, after recent surgery and the inactivity that followed, my weight crept up and my digestion slowed down. Not that I like chatting about it, but I began to have constipation and bloating issues. Thankfully, I bid adieu to my newly obtained belly pooch and GI complaints during this innovative 3-week plan. I learned how to avoid all the surprising Belly Bullies causing my tummy woes, and how to enjoy the yummy Belly Buddies that helped me shrink and soothe. I've been trouble-free ever since!

A bonus? I slept like a baby while eating this new way. I wasn't the only one. Rob McMahon noticed how refreshed he felt when he woke up in the morning, after only one full day on the diet! Another tester, Jonathan Bigham, noted that he no longer needed to set his alarm to wake up. And this specific combination of high magnesium, low sugar, high-fiber, and carb-light foods even seemed to make my hair grow faster!

No need to deprive yourself by eating tasteless foods to keep your tummy calm and symptom free. The notion that everyone with digestive issues should eat a bland and boring diet is simply unfounded. In fact, adherents to the 21-Day Tummy plan enjoy a variety of flavorful foods and a calmer belly.

We all loved the foods and recipes on the 21-Day Tummy plan. Since they were so popular, I created this cookbook to provide even more mouthwatering, tummy-taming recipes. I know you will not be disappointed. You'll never get bored with the vast selection of recipes you'll find in this cookbook, from energizing breakfasts, savory soups, delectable salads, filling main entrees, and even sweet but healthy treats—all created with ingredients that shrink and calm tummies. These recipes make eating well a no-brainer because they automatically cut out Belly Bullies and pack in Belly Buddies.

Best of all for the busiest among us? Most of these recipes can be prepared with less than 30 minutes of hands-on time. They are easy to prepare, and many can be frozen ahead for easy grab-and-go meals during a hectic workweek.

If you had success with the 21-Day Tummy plan, then this cookbook will provide more tasty inspirations to keep you going. If you're new to *21-Day Tummy Diet*, this cookbook will provide the major highlights of the original book so you, too, can start calming and shrinking your belly *right now!*

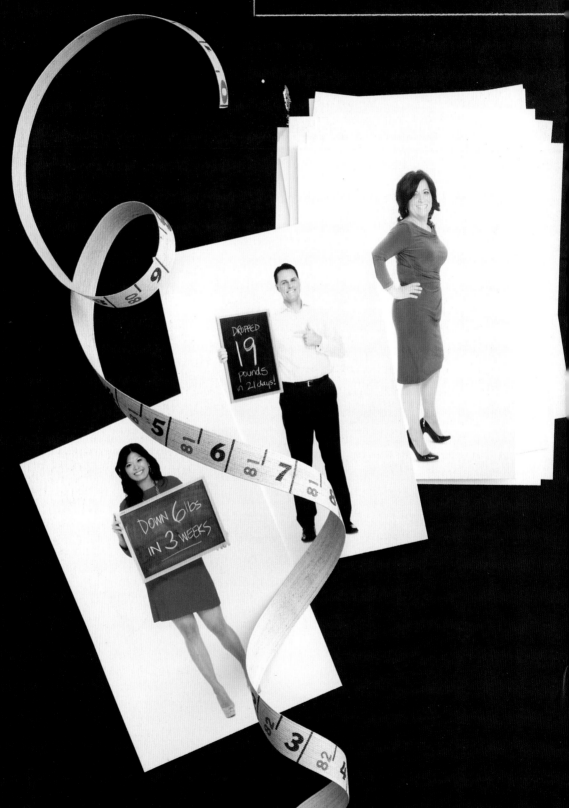

DROPPED
19
pounds
in 21 days!

DOWN 6 lbs
IN 3 WEEKS

Chapter 1

Tummy Troubles Begone!

Banish belly bulges, bloating, heartburn, and more

According to the Harvard School of Public Health, 200 million adult men and almost 300 million adult women in the world are obese.[1] The United States has the highest level of obesity worldwide. More than a third of American adults are obese, and nearly 70 percent are overweight.[2, 3] And, to their dismay, on many people the extra pounds seem to accumulate around their tummy. Not only is that belly fat unsightly, it's also deadly. Visceral fat deep under your skin smothers your abdominal organs and secretes hormones and other substances that contribute to heart disease, type 2 diabetes, cancer, and many other serious health conditions.

> To their dismay, on many people the extra pounds all seem to accumulate around their tummy.

Along with the extra weight come other tummy troubles. Even subtle weight gain ups the chances for GI problems, not to mention that uncomfortable feeling when your favorite jeans feel tight. According to a study in the *New England Journal of Medicine,* even in women with a normal body mass index (BMI), when their BMI increased by just 3.5, they were more likely to experience frequent acid reflux.[4] So it's no surprise that the prevalence of digestive disorders has grown along with our waistlines. The occurrence of weekly heartburn, for instance, rose nearly 50 percent over the last decade.[5]

According to the U.S. Department of Health and Human Services' National Institutes of Health, 60 million to 70 million people in the United States are affected by digestive diseases.[6] Among the most common: gas and bloating, heartburn and acid reflux, constipation, diarrhea, and irritable bowel syndrome (IBS). Researchers from the University of North Carolina, Chapel Hill found in a recent study that 65 percent of respondents surveyed by phone rated their gastrointestinal symptoms as moderate or severe in intensity, which disrupted their normal activities.[7]

A two-for-one diet, the 21-Day Tummy eating plan takes aim at both types of tummy troubles simultaneously so that your stomach slims and calms down right away.

The Links Between Weight and Digestion

In researching and writing *21-Day Tummy Diet,* I uncovered a connection between weight gain and digestive issues that hadn't yet hit the national news. Trillions of bacteria live in our intestines, and scientists are just beginning to understand how maintaining the right balance of these microbes can keep our tummies happy. In addition, chronic inflammation adds to our big bellies and triggers our digestive woes.

Unbalanced Gut Bacteria

Conventional wisdom says that the key to weight management is a balance between calories consumed and calories burned by your body. But reality is a bit more complicated.

A recent Mayo Clinic study revealed that the "bacterial flora of obese mice and humans include fewer Bacteroidetes and correspondingly more Firmicutes [two of the main types of microbes to inhabit the GI tract] than that of their lean counterparts, suggesting that differences in caloric extraction for ingested food substance may be due to the composition of the gut microbiota," the microbes that inhabit your intestine.[8] Excessive amounts of Firmicutes promote fat storage. By breaking normally indigestible fiber into absorbable short-chain fatty acids, our gut bacteria make extra calories out of the food we eat. How generous (not)!

In a series of experiments done at Washington University of Medicine, researchers found that, despite eating more, mice free of any gut bacteria had a lower body fat content compared to conventionally raised mice. The gut bacteria from the normal mice were then transplanted into the bacteria-free mice. Within 2 weeks, these mice gained 60 percent more body fat, without changing how they ate or exercised. They also developed insulin resistance (a precursor to diabetes) and had increased levels of the hunger hormone leptin. Even their fat cells got larger.[9]

Gut bacteria may even change our metabolism. After gastric bypass surgery, patients see a rapid and sustained increase of *Escherichia* and *Akkermansia*. At the same time, their metabolism speeds up and their weight and body fat drop rapidly.[10]

Besides making us fatter, our gut bacteria can throw a wrench into our digestive system. A study recently published in the *American Journal of Gastroenterology* found that kids with irritable bowel syndrome have fewer bifidobacteria, among other differences in gut flora, than normal healthy kids. Researchers think these bacteria alterations may cause the diarrhea that these children are prone to.[11] Another study shows that an increase in gram-negative bacteria (that is, bacteria that share characteristics linked with disease) in the esophagus coincides with inflammation and cell changes that are commonly seen in gastroesophageal reflux (GERD).[12]

Changes in your gut bacteria don't just affect your digestive system. Bacterial shifts have been linked with autism, rheumatoid arthritis, heart disease, and even cancer. And the scientific community is just beginning to connect the dots between our gut microbes and our health and well-being.

It's important to note that not all bacteria are bad news. Gut bacteria help break down our food for digestion, creating vitamin B and vitamin K to keep our body healthy and strong. Plus, some reduce the risk of certain diseases, including cancer and allergies, and help repel infections and toxins.

Unfortunately, staying healthy isn't as simple as getting more good bacteria and getting rid of the bad bacteria. Most microbes can both help and harm you, depending on how much you have and how sensitive your system is. For instance, having too few Firmicutes is linked with inflammatory bowel disease, while hosting too many of these bacteria is linked with obesity.[13] It's all about balance.

Inflammation That Won't Stop

Inflammation is not inherently a bad thing. It's a protective reaction, our body's way of ridding itself of infections to help us heal. Our immune system kicks into high gear, fighting infectious pathogens with a burst of immune activity to repair and nourish wounds. But when inflammation goes rogue and spirals out of control, it can impact every cell in our body.

This type of chronic inflammation can actually make you fat. Whole body inflammation is a predictor of future weight gain.[14] Our body attempts to defend itself from inflammation by producing anti-inflammatory chemicals. Unfortunately, these chemicals interfere with the normal function of the hormone leptin. Normally, leptin tells your brain to stop eating when you are full. But, if you have chronic inflammation, your brain doesn't get the message. That means you still feel hungry (even after you've just finished a meal) so you keep eating. This leads to weight gain.

> When inflammation goes rogue and spirals out of control, it can impact *every* cell in our body.

And, in a vicious cycle, weight gain causes even more inflammation. In a paper published in March 2013, researchers found that when you overfeed your fat cells, they produce a group of proteins that usually only appear to help your body fight off a bacterial or viral infection. In essence, they are initiating a false alarm, but your immune system reacts as if the danger was real and responds with inflammation.[15] In another recent study, 11 healthy men and three women were fed 1.4 times their calorie needs for 8 weeks. Researchers concluded the participants developed enlarged fat cells and greater amounts of visceral fat. The visceral fat released substances called cytokines and chemokines, which trigger an inflammatory response, raise blood sugar and cholesterol levels, and increase blood pressure.[16] This increases your risk for heart disease, type 2 diabetes, and even more weight gain.

Inflammation can occur anywhere in your body, and along with inflammation often comes pain. Any condition with an "–itis" at the end of it refers to inflammation—think about arthritis, bursitis, tendonitis, or rhinitis, all conditions marked by painful swelling. In your GI tract, inflammation can flare up in your esophagus (esophagitis), stomach (gastritis), and intestines (colitis). These and other inflammatory conditions in the gut have all been linked with bacterial imbalances. Gastritis often follows an *H. pylori* infection. GERD, Crohn's, and ulcerative colitis sufferers have alterations in their gut bacteria, too. Compared to healthy individuals, for instance, people with ulcerative colitis have more gram-negative bacteria and fewer healthy *Lactobacillus* and *Akkermansia*.[17]

What's Fueling Inflammation and Microbial Imbalance

Scientists have been studying chronic inflammation for decades, so we have a good idea of what causes it. Stress, exposure to environmental toxins, repeated infections, and weight gain all fan the flames. So do some gut microbes. What we eat is the biggest culprit: The standard Western diet, supersized with unhealthy fats and refined carbs but lacking many critical nutrients, is a prescription for chronic inflammation.

While researchers have known about gut microbes for just as long, though, they have only recently begun to understand how widespread the impact of these tiny organisms really is. Mapping the number and types of gut bacteria in humans, identifying how they affect different diseases, and figuring out what foods or habits can change the makeup of each individual's microbiota are all subjects of ongoing studies. This is very new science, so our understanding of this complex system changes every day. That being said, there are some things we do know

(continued on page 8)

Rob McMahon, Age 42

**LOST 19 POUNDS and
2 ½ BELLY INCHES in 21 days!**

At 6'3", Rob is tall enough to carry his weight well. Most of his colleagues (me included!) were surprised to learn that he had extra pounds to lose—but at 233 pounds, his BMI put him on the high end of the "over-weight" category.

Plus, he had constant, severe heartburn. He had been relying on daily prescription medication to control the symptoms and, previously, when he had tried to wean himself off of it, as soon as he skipped a dose, he felt a lot of discomfort. But on day one of the 21-Day Tummy diet, "I stopped taking the medication, and I did not need it once. My acid reflux is completely gone." Amazing!

No more daily heartburn medication!

Rob's goal had been to "start the journey of losing 15 pounds," but he didn't necessarily expect to do it all in 21 days. Instead, he blew away his expectations, dropping a whopping 19 pounds—that's almost a pound a day! "To know that I lost even more than I wanted . . . I just simply feel better about myself."

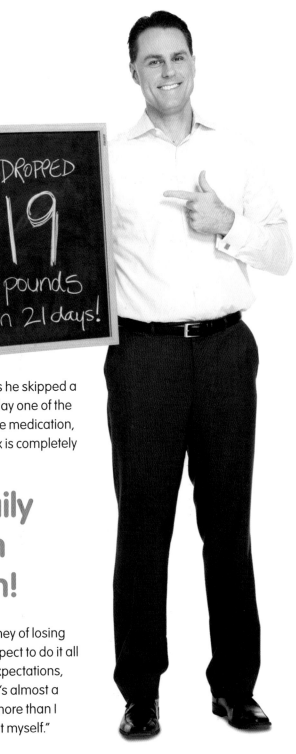

(continued from page 6)

for sure about what affects our gut bacteria—and it turns out to look a lot like the list of things that cause chronic inflammation: stress, infections, changes in weight, and our diet.

To create the 21-Day Tummy plan, Kate and I paired the newest discoveries about the foods that contribute to chronic inflammation and imbalances in gut bacteria—most notably, carb-dense and rapidly fermentable foods—together with time-tested knowledge about pro- and anti-inflammatory fats and the effects of magnesium.

Carb Density

Refined or unrefined. High glycemic or low glycemic. Starchy or nonstarchy. Over the years, as researchers have been working to tease out the differences between various types of carbs and what effects they have in the human body, dieters have been trying to figure out which ones will really help them lose weight and which will cause them to gain.

But while all of these distinctions have helped us learn more about how carbs affect our health, none of them quite explain the paradox of the Kitavan Islanders. These Melanesian people eat a diet that is about 60 to 70 percent carbohydrate, including many starchy foods such as sweet potatoes and bananas that are high-glycemic—that is, they break down into sugars quickly, which is thought to contribute to type 2 diabetes and other health problems. But they have lower blood sugar, insulin, and leptin levels than Westerners—and almost no cases of overweight, diabetes, and atherosclerosis (hardening of the arteries, which can lead to heart disease).[18, 19, 20]

How is this possible? Ian Spreadbury, a researcher from the Gastrointestinal Diseases Research Unit at Queen's University in Ontario, Canada, proposed that carb density is the issue. The foods the Kitavan Islanders eat—which he calls ancestral foods—all have a low carb density. That is, they have low levels of carbohydrates compared to the weight of the food (as measured in grams). The average banana, for instance, weighs about 125 grams (minus the peel). Some of that weight, though, comes from the moisture packed in the banana and some from non-digestible fibers. The non-fibrous carbs we actually digest make up a little less than 30 grams, or about 23 percent of the weight. Moreover, these carbs are stored in cells that don't appear to break down until after stomach acids and other digestive juices start in on them. That not only keeps the calories we get from bananas and other ancestral foods proportionately lower than from other foods of the same weight but also means they are less likely to contribute to inflammation.

The Western diet, by contrast, includes a lot of processed foods made with flour and sugar. These "modern" foods, such as breads, cakes, and pasta, are very high in carb density. More than 80 percent of the weight of a pretzel, for instance, is carbohydrate. And, thanks to the milling of the flour, pretzels lack intact cell walls. So the carbs in pretzels are released into your digestive system as soon as you take a bite. Flooding your stomach and small intestine with carbs upsets the balance of gut bacteria and produces "an inflammatory microbiota via the upper intestinal tract, with dietary fat able to effect a 'double hit' by increasing systemic absorption of lipopolysaccharide."[21] Lipopolysaccharide (LPS), a molecule on the outer part of gram-negative bacteria, is a toxin that can also trigger an inflammatory response.

> Kitavan Islanders eat a diet that is 60 to 70 percent carbohydrates but have almost no cases of overweight, diabetes, and atherosclerosis.

Because carb-dense foods contribute to both chronic inflammation and microbial imbalance, the 21-Day Tummy plan minimizes them, drastically reducing processed and refined sugars as well as most grains.

Rapidly Fermentable Carbs, or FODMAPs

Besides being carb-dense, many modern processed foods contain a type of carbohydrate—rapidly fermentable carbs, or FODMAPs—that can make our bellies very unhappy. Our bodies either lack the enzymes needed to digest these carbs or don't absorb them efficiently, allowing them to pass through to our large intestine. Here, bacteria ferment them, breaking them down into acids, which combine to create gas. When we eat too many of these rapidly fermentable carbs, we experience a buildup of gas, which can cause uncomfortable bloating or flatulence or contribute to constipation. FODMAPs also draw water into the intestine, which can cause diarrhea or cramping.

Rapidly fermentable carbs may upset the balance of gut bacteria by overfeeding them. They may also lead to inflammation via toxins produced by the bacteria they feed.

There are several different types of rapidly fermentable carbs, as indicated by the acronym by which they are known—**FODMAPs.** This stands for:

> **F**ermentable
> **O**ligosaccharides: fructans and
>   galacto-oligosaccharides
> **D**isaccharides: lactose
> **M**onosaccharides: fructose
> **A**nd
> **P**olyols: sugar alcohols such as sorbitol, mannitol, maltitol, and xylitol

Don't be fooled by the fancy scientific names; FODMAPs may lurk in a number of common foods, like beans, milk, honey, apples, and cauliflower. (You can find a fuller list in Appendix B.) Because they can easily throw your gut flora out of whack, Kate and I have classified all FODMAPs as Belly Bullies and have taken them all off the table during your 21-Day Tummy plan. However, please note that you don't necessarily need or want to avoid them all completely and forever.

People react differently to different FODMAPs. During the plan, for instance, I discovered that my tummy was especially sensitive to fructose, so much so that even a couple teaspoons of agave nectar (which is more than 80 percent fructose) sent me home early with a stomachache. Tester Dorothy Nuzzo, on the other hand, had no trouble with fructose, but found that any time she ate onions, bread, and other foods high in fructans, her heartburn and bloating "came back big time."

This can happen for a variety of reasons. Some people may lack a specific digestive enzyme, as in lactose intolerance. Due to genetics, some individuals may not be equipped to digest fructose efficiently. Others may have too many bacteria in the small intestine, a condition known as small intestinal bacterial overgrowth (SIBO); these bacteria ferment FODMAPs in the narrow small intestine, which can contribute to pain and cramping. And, of course, which and how many bacteria live in your gut—the balance of your gut microbiome—can affect how you react to a FODMAP. How many FODMAPs you consume can also make a difference in how your tummy reacts. The more FODMAPs you eat at one time, the more likely you are to experience digestive symptoms.

Many foods containing FODMAPs, though, are otherwise healthy (such as blackberries and snow peas), so avoiding them if you are not sensitive to them simply doesn't make sense. After 21 days, when your tummy is trim and calm, try the Belly

ALL ABOUT FIBER

Fiber, the indigestible part of plant foods, comes in many shapes and forms. The 21-Day Tummy plan reduces the rapidly fermentable types (also called FODMAPs) known to contribute to excess gas, bloating, and other GI symptoms.

The right kinds of fiber, though, are critical to good digestion; they add bulk to our stool and aid regular elimination. Most Americans fall short of the 25 to 38 grams of fiber recommended by the Institute of Medicine. The 21-Day Tummy diet incorporates an average of 25 grams of low-FODMAP fiber per day into the plan to keep your belly full and satisfied and keep your digestive tract in tip-top working order. Fiber supplements can provide an extra boost of fiber, but beware! Some fiber supplements are made with FODMAPs, so they may actually bother your tummy. Fiber should come from food first to provide extra perks—namely, vitamins, minerals, antioxidants, and disease-fighting phytochemicals, not to mention taste!

Bully Tests found in Appendix A on page 292. You'll learn which FODMAPs trigger your digestive symptoms (your *personal* Belly Bullies) and which you can add back to your new healthy diet—and in what amounts. I had suspected I was becoming lactose intolerant when my daily tall glasses of milk started making my tummy grumble, and I was right. But Kate explained that this didn't mean I had to swear off all dairy foods forever. Through the 21-Day Tummy plan, I learned that I could snack on Greek yogurt and hard cheeses (both relatively low in lactose) without fear, and I could even enjoy the occasional cup of milk while remaining symptom free.

The science of FODMAPs is relatively new, and food testing to determine the FODMAP content of various foods is ongoing, mostly at Monash University in Melbourne, Australia. As we learn more about the content of these fermentable sugars in different foods, the low FODMAP diet guidelines will continue to be updated and refined. Plus, your tolerance to FODMAPs can change over time, as you balance your gut bacteria. So if you find that most of the Belly Bullies give you trouble, give yourself another month or two of 21-Day Tummy eating, then try the Belly Bully Tests again.

Pro-Inflammatory Fats

Among the biggest triggers of inflammation are three types of dietary fat: trans fats, saturated fats, and omega-6 fats. Trans fats can be found in some foods naturally (milk and beef), but the majority of these dangerous fats are man-made during a process called hydrogenation, where liquid oils are bombarded with hydrogen molecules. Trans fats damage the inner lining of our blood vessels, inflaming them and potentially leading to blood clots.[22]

The gut microbiota of people who consume a lot of saturated fatty acids (found in red meat and dairy foods) contain predominantly gram-negative bacteria rich in the toxin

(continued on page 14)

Tonya Carkeet, Age 32

**LOST 6 POUNDS and
4 BELLY INCHES IN 21 DAYS!**

Weight has been a struggle for Tonya Carkeet her whole life. While she would lose a few pounds here and there, they always came back—and then some, especially after she endured a difficult pregnancy and the delivery of her daughter, Trista. Her weight ballooned to a high of 280 pounds, and at that weight, she says, "something always hurt." Tonya suffered from constant muscle aches, severe heartburn, diarrhea, and stomach pains, and her blood sugar was near diabetic levels. By the time Trista turned 2, Tonya was finding it exhausting to keep up with her. Plus, "Trista is the first grandbaby in the family, and everywhere we went, there were always cameras. I would literally hide from them."

Setting an Example by Slimming Down

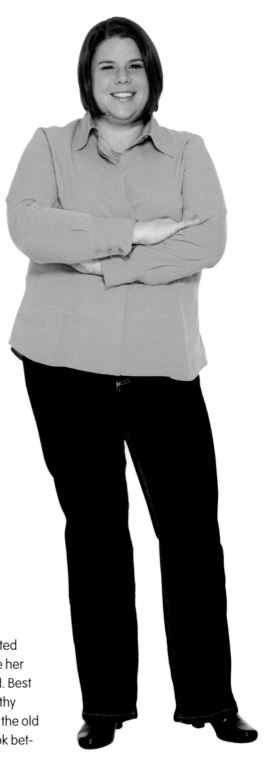

After the 21-Day Tummy plan, her digestive problems were completely gone. An unexpected bonus? Her feelings of depression lifted, while her optimism, energy, and self-confidence soared. Best of all was seeing Trista learn to love new, healthy foods. "It's hard to believe I was content to live the old way for so long," Tonya says. "I feel better, I look better, and the future is much brighter."

(continued from page 12)

lipopolysaccharide (LPS). When receptors in the cell membranes detect LPS, they activate enzymes that lead to insulin resistance. At the same time, when these receptors detect saturated fats, they trigger an inflammatory reaction.[23] Trans fats and saturated fats also raise your risk for heart disease, type 2 diabetes, and obesity.

As if that weren't enough, studies show that Americans are now consuming 14 to 25 times more omega-6 fats than omega-3 fats, mostly through corn and soybean oils used in crackers, breads, and other packaged foods. While both of these types of unsaturated fats are essential for good health, it's important to keep them in better balance: The lower the ratio, the lower your risk for health issues. People who eat more omega-6 than omega-3 fats not only have more inflammatory markers called cytokines (proteins that regulate inflammatory response) but also are at greater risk for depression.[24]

Luckily, just as trans fats, saturated fats, and omega-6 fats turn on inflammation, other types of fat turn it off. One of the key tenets of the 21-Day Tummy plan is to eat more anti-inflammatory fats, which include omega-3 fats and, my favorite, monounsaturated fats (MUFAs).

Magnesium Deficiency

Given all you hear about Americans eating too much, it may surprise you to learn that malnutrition is common in the United States. Despite the abundance of food on our shelves, much of it is lacking in vitamins, minerals, and other vital nutrients. One such nutrient is magnesium. Among American adults, 68 percent consumed less than the recommended daily amount of magnesium, according to researchers at the Medical University of South Carolina.[25] Canadians are little better. More than one-third of 19- to 30-year-olds fall short on magnesium intake, and the incidence increases with age: More than 60 percent of the 71-year-old and older

MEET THE BELLY BULLIES

We've identified the foods most likely to cause belly fat, bloating, indigestion, and other tummy troubles. These are foods that are high in carb density and FODMAPs—most are also low in magnesium, and implicated in inflammation. We call them the Belly Bullies, and you'll want to avoid them during your 21-Day Tummy plan:

- **Carb-dense foods** (refined carbs and grains): white flour, sugar
- **Pro-inflammatory fats** (trans fats, saturated fats, omega-6 fats): red meat, processed foods, fast food, full-fat cheese, fatty processed meats like salami and bologna
- **High-lactose foods:** milk, regular yogurt
- **High-fructose foods:** high-fructose corn syrup, honey, agave nectar, mangoes, apples, pears
- **High-fructan foods:** wheat, garlic, onions and relatives (leeks, shallots), chicory root extract (inulin)
- **High-GOS (galacto-oligosaccharide) foods:** beans/legumes, especially red kidney beans and soybeans
- **High-polyol foods:** artificial sugars, plums, prunes, apricots, nectarines, blackberries, mushrooms, cauliflower, sugar-free mints and gum

You may be surprised to find so many fruits and vegetables on this list. Remember that many foods high in FODMAPs are healthy, and that sensitivity varies from person to person. So after your 21 days, you may want to add some of these foods back in limited quantities; in Appendix A, we'll explain how to determine which ones specifically bother you. (If you have an especially sensitive tummy, check out the fuller list of Belly Bullies in Appendix B so you know what to steer clear of.)

crowd does not consume enough of this important nutrient.[26]

This is simply bad news. Poor magnesium intake is associated with health issues ranging from migraine headaches, Alzheimer's disease, recurrent bacterial infections, kidney and liver damage, premenstrual syndrome, and calcium deficiency (which can contribute to mood swings and osteoporosis).[27]

Researchers have found a link between low-magnesium diets and elevated C-reactive protein, a marker of inflammation in the body. Magnesium deficiency, especially when combined with a high-fructose diet, also causes insulin resistance (a precursor to type 2 diabetes) along with high blood pressure, high triglyceride levels, and chronic inflammation.[28] This important mineral also helps our muscles and nerves function properly and even helps keep our bones strong.

The 21-Day Tummy plan fights back by emphasizing foods high in magnesium, such as spinach, brown rice, quinoa, oat bran, pumpkin seeds, and peanuts.

Relief from Five Digestive Disasters

By minimizing Belly Bullies and piling on Belly Buddies—the foods that can reduce inflammation and bring our gut bacteria into balance (you'll learn more about these delicious healing foods in Chapter 2)—the 21-Day Tummy diet helps you shed dangerous belly fat. Not only that, the plan can also prevent, alleviate, and sometimes even cure five digestive disorders:

1. Gas and bloating
2. Heartburn and acid reflux
3. Constipation
4. Diarrhea
5. Irritable bowel syndrome (IBS)

In designing the 21-Day Tummy plan, Kate and I chose to focus on these five conditions because they are the most common (63 million North Americans suffer from chronic constipation, while 65 million report acid reflux at least once a week) [29, 30] and because their causes are similar enough that one diet could treat them all. These stomach problems are bothersome in and of themselves. Even worse, they can signal or develop into more serious diseases like hemorrhoids, dehydration, esophageal cancer, or colon cancer.

If you suffer from other GI issues, like inflammatory bowel disease (such as ulcerative colitis or Crohn's disease), gallstones, or peptic ulcers, talk to your doctor before trying the 21-Day Tummy plan. The diet may help relieve some of your symptoms, but you need an individualized treatment plan managed by a health care provider. If you have celiac disease or are gluten intolerant, it's easy to make the 21-Day Tummy diet gluten free. If you are lactose intolerant, this diet was made for you.

Gas and Bloating

Foods that are not absorbed well by your body, such as fiber and FODMAPs, become food for our intestinal bacteria. When these gut microbes ferment these undigested food components, they give off gas. A little gas is okay, but if you eat too much of these foods and your bacteria are out of balance, you wind up with excess gas, which you may release as burping or flatulence.

When gas is trapped in your stomach or small intestine, due to a sluggish digestive tract, you'll feel an uncomfortable bloating in your abdomen. If your intestine is particularly sensitive, you may experience cramping and pain. Trapped gas is common in conditions such as irritable bowel syndrome (IBS).

By minimizing the FODMAPs that our bacteria love so much, the 21-Day Tummy diet reduces gas production and prevents bloating.

Heartburn and Acid Reflux

When you swallow, your lower esophageal sphincter, a circular band of muscle around the bottom part of the esophagus, relaxes, allowing food and fluids to enter your stomach. After the food enters your stomach, your esophageal sphincter closes again. If it doesn't close properly, partially digested food and liquid, along with stomach acid, can seep back up into your esophagus. This is acid reflux, and it causes heartburn, a burning sensation in your chest. (Ouch, it hurts just thinking about this!)

If you suffer from acid reflux more than twice a week on a regular basis, you may have GERD, or gastro-esophageal reflux disease. A chronic digestive disorder, GERD may lead to inflammation of the esophagus. These regular episodes of the surge of stomach acid into the esophagus can lead to scarring and a more dangerous condition known at Barrett's esophagus, a disease linked with esophageal cancer risk. If acid reflux troubles you, be sure to visit your doctor.

Acid reflux and GERD appear to be growing problems. According to a 2011 Norwegian study, the number of people reporting symptoms of acid reflux at least once a week escalated from 31 percent in 1995 to 40 percent by 2009.[31] I bet they could all benefit from the 21-Day Tummy, which cuts down on the fried and fatty foods that can frequently trigger heartburn.

Constipation

Constipation impacts almost everyone at some point, but women and the elderly are most likely to have a chronic problem. If you have two or fewer bowel movements in a week, or experience straining, hard stools, or incomplete evacuation more than 25 percent of the time for at least 3 months, you are considered constipated.[32]

Constipation occurs when your bowels are sluggish. Lack of fluids, inadequate fiber, stress, and any number of other things can cause it. Interestingly, but no surprise, our gut bacteria may play a role. Methane-producing bacteria are associated with slowing down the bowel, likely contributing to constipation.[33] These same microbes are also associated with a higher body mass index.[34]

With its assortment of fiber-rich foods, including chia, flax, and pumpkin seeds, the 21-Day Tummy diet worked wonders for my constipation problem, and I know it will work for you!

No one likes to feel "backed up." The diet will flatten your bloat and clean your system, perhaps scrubbing it of those methane-producing, constipation-causing microbes!

Diarrhea

Loose, watery stools that occur more frequently than usual, sometimes accompanied by abdominal cramps—that's diarrhea. Acute diarrhea, usually caused by an infection or food-borne illness, comes on suddenly and lasts just a few days. Chronic diarrhea, on the other hand, may last more than 4 weeks and can indicate a serious disorder, such as inflammatory bowel disease (ulcerative colitis or Crohn's disease) or irritable bowel syndrome.

Food intolerances—when your body doesn't digest a specific nutrient properly—are also common causes of chronic diarrhea. Lactose, fructose, and other FODMAPs are often poorly absorbed, while gluten, a protein found in wheat, barley, and rye, can damage the small intestine. These rapidly fermentable sugars and fibers are known to draw water into the colon, where it makes your stools more watery, thus contributing to diarrhea in sensitive individuals.[35] The 21-Day Tummy diet removes these and other foods associated with diarrhea.

Irritable bowel syndrome (IBS)

Irritable bowel syndrome (IBS) is an intestinal motility disorder. That means your large intestine either moves too slow, causing constipa-

WHEN DIARRHEA IS DANGEROUS

If you experience any of the following symptoms, see your doctor immediately:

- Acute diarrhea that lasts more than 2 days
- Blood in the stool (bright red or black stools)
- Pain moving your bowels
- Diarrhea accompanied by a fever
- Signs of dehydration (such as headaches, fatigue, irritability, inability to concentrate, dry lips, thirst, dark yellow urine)

If you are experiencing diarrhea or show any signs of dehydration, be sure to drink eight or more 8-ounce glasses of water per day along with some electrolyte-containing beverages, such as coconut water.

tion, or too fast, causing diarrhea. Plus, because the nerves and muscles of your large intestine aren't working efficiently, they can trap gas, causing bloating. Those with IBS also have what is known as visceral hypersensitivity. This refers to an exaggerated pain sensation in the intestines.[36] IBS is estimated to impact one in five Americans, and those who suffer with IBS are three times more likely to call in sick. Talk about a life-disrupting disorder![37]

IBS can be tough to diagnose because other medical conditions can mimic its symptoms. These include:

- Lactose intolerance, in which individuals can't digest the lactose in dairy products

- Celiac disease, an autoimmune condition in which gluten damages the intestinal lining

- Small intestinal bacterial overgrowth (SIBO), in which bacteria that normally reside in the large intestine creep up into the small intestine

Scientists still aren't sure exactly what causes IBS, but a group at Australia's Monash University has some clues on how to manage it. They're the folks who identified the rapidly fermentable carbs, or FODMAPs, we learned about earlier, and it appears that FODMAPs may be the culprit behind many IBS symptoms. About 76 percent of IBS sufferers who try a low-FODMAP diet experience significant relief from their symptoms.[42]

Similarly, the 21-Day Tummy plan carefully pulls out these troubling FODMAPs to keep IBS symptoms at bay. But it adds inflammation-zapping nutrients such as magnesium, MUFAs, and omega-3 fats along with select (non-gassy) fiber-rich foods to keep your digestive system humming.

✳✳✳

Sometimes it's challenging to let go of old habits. Grabbing snacks at the gas station on your way home from work. Ordering fries or chips on the side. Wanting a healthier body is one thing, making the lifelong changes so it will happen is another. But I promise that if you make the healthy changes in the 21-Day Tummy plan, you'll feel the best you have in years. The best part? This plan is so full of delicious and filling foods, you won't even feel like you are on a diet.

It's time to get your health in check and learn how to eat in a way that will keep you lean and clean for a lifetime! Get ready to cook up some Belly Buddies!

ABOUT CELIAC DISEASE AND GLUTEN INTOLERANCE

Celiac disease is an autoimmune disorder, a severe form of food hypersensitivity, in which gluten—a protein found in wheat, barley, and rye—damages the lining of the small intestine. Although researchers are unable to pinpoint exactly why, celiac disease is on the rise in the United States.[39] Symptoms of celiac disease range from person to person. While some have silent celiac (suffering intestinal damage but no GI symptoms), others may experience nausea, gas, bloating, diarrhea, constipation, heartburn, fatigue, skin rashes, and even neurological problems.

In non-celiac gluten sensitivity, also known as gluten intolerance, gluten does not affect the intestinal lining but sufferers still experience many of the same symptoms. The Center for Celiac Research at the University of Maryland reports that approximately 18 million Americans suffer from gluten intolerance.[40]

Both conditions are treated by removing sources of gluten from the diet. The 21-Day Tummy diet removes most gluten sources; the trace amounts that may be left are well tolerated by most people with gluten sensitivity but can cause serious problems for people with celiac disease. For this reason, ingredients that may be contaminated with gluten are called out in the recipes so you can avoid them if necessary. (Potential culprits include Greek yogurt, oats, chia seeds, soy sauce, baking powder, broth, spice blends, mustard, spreadable cheese, and seasoned nuts and seeds.)

If you suspect you may have celiac disease, please get tested before you begin the 21-Day Tummy diet. Celiac disease is usually first diagnosed with a blood test to detect antibodies to gluten; if you've been off gluten for a while, as you will be on this plan, your test results are likely to be skewed.

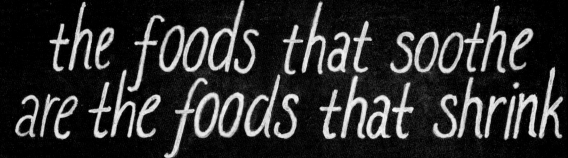

the foods that soothe
are the foods that shrink

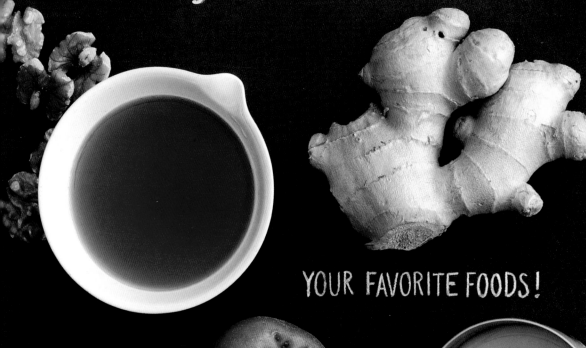

YOUR FAVORITE FOODS!

VERSATILE AND FLAVORFUL

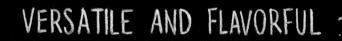

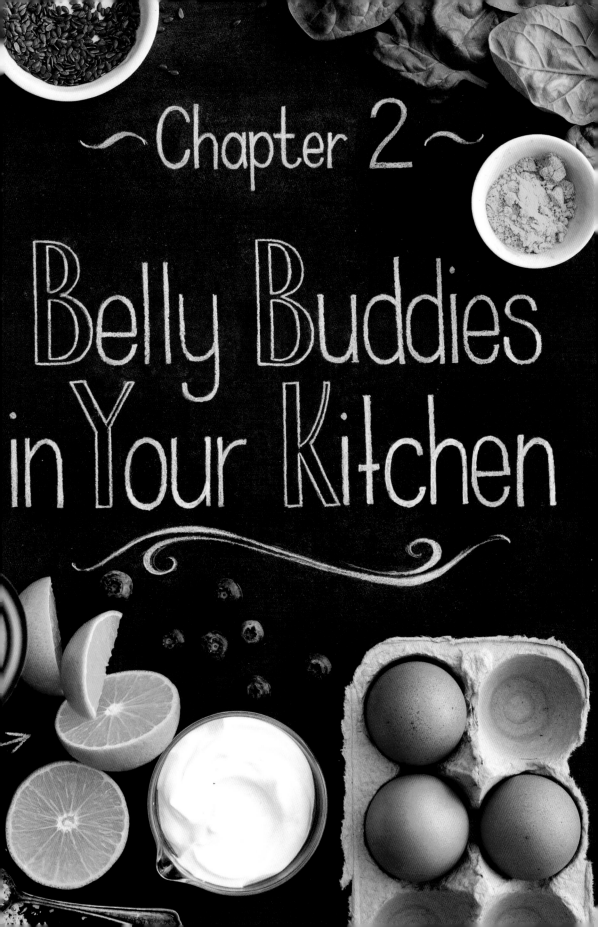

~Chapter 2~

Belly Buddies in Your Kitchen

For many of us, it's a fact of life: If we bring it home, we will eat it. Stash a bag of chocolate chip cookies in the cupboard and, yes, they will be gobbled up. Cook up a delicious dinner meal and that too will be devoured. Contrary to popular belief, healthy foods don't have to be boring, nor should they be! Plain broiled chicken may sound like a snore, but how about Chicken Mac and Cheese or Chicken Enchiladas? Perhaps Tofu Coconut Curry or Margarita Shrimp Salad gets your mouth watering. That's only a sample of the delectable recipes in the *21-Day Tummy Diet Cookbook*, which includes a variety of belly-friendly and fat-slashing breakfast, lunch, and dinner recipes. Don't worry, we included desserts, too!

> Contrary to popular belief, healthy foods don't have to be boring, nor should they be!

All of the recipes have been carefully crafted to exclude the bothersome Belly Bullies that disrupt our gut bacteria and cause chronic inflammation. As we ditch the Belly Bullies, we want to add some buddies that pick us up when we feel down. Belly Buddies are foods that minimize inflammation and balance our gut bacteria to soothe, calm, and flatten our tummies. They are low in FODMAPs, so they help minimize gas, bloating, and bathroom troubles. They are also carb-light—that is, they are carbs as you would find them in nature: strawberries from a bush, not strawberry jam; a potato from the ground, not potato flakes in a box. Simply put, Belly Buddies include foods *plucked off a plant, not made in a plant*. Belly Buddies are inflammation busters, rich in magnesium, omega-3s, and monounsaturated fats (MUFAs). They are high in fiber, which helps keep your blood sugar steady and your large intestine working at its prime.

Belly Buddies satisfy our cravings, too. From sweet strawberries to creamy peanut butter to hearty oats, they include some of your favorite foods; others may become your new favorite pals.

Without further delay, say hello to your **Belly Buddies:**

1. **High-fiber and antioxidant-rich vegetables,** especially kale, Swiss chard, and spinach; also green beans, bean sprouts, bok choy, carrots, cucumbers, eggplant, endive, lettuce, parsnips, turnips, tomatoes, zucchini, and potatoes

2. **Balanced-fructose fruits,** especially bananas and blueberries; also grapes, oranges, strawberries, kiwis, pineapple, papaya, cantaloupe, honeydew, raspberries, and star fruit

3. **Low-FODMAP, high-fiber grains,** especially oats, brown rice, and quinoa; also buckwheat, polenta, and rice bran

4. **Nuts and nut butters,** especially peanuts and walnuts

5. **Seeds,** especially chia, pumpkin, and flax

6. **Healthy fats** (omega-3s, MUFAs): salmon, mackerel, tuna, herring, sardines, flaxseeds and flaxseed oil, olives and olive oil, and canola oil

7. **Lean protein:** fish and seafood, poultry, lean cuts of beef and pork, eggs

8. **Greek yogurt**

9. **Coconut milk**

10. **Ginger**

11. **Turmeric**

12. **Maple syrup**

Let's take a closer look at the Belly Buddies and some simple ways to make the most of them.

Belly Buddy #1: High-Fiber and Antioxidant-Rich Vegetables

Vegetables make up the largest category of Belly Buddies, and for good reason. Plucked straight from the plant, fresh produce is brimming with fiber, vitamins, minerals, and other important nutrients—including anti-inflammatory magnesium. A few otherwise healthy vegetables, though, such as onions and cauliflower, contain FODMAPs that can lead to gas and bloating. So Kate and I carefully selected vegetables that could soothe inflammation while keeping your digestive tract humming. Leafy green vegetables like kale, Swiss chard, and spinach are especially high in anti-inflammatory magnesium and other antioxidants.

HIGH-FIBER, ANTIOXIDANT-RICH VEGGIES

Arugula

Bean sprouts

Bell peppers (all varieties, including green, red, yellow, and orange)

Bok choy

Cabbage (red and green only; savoy and napa are limited)

Carrots

Celery root (celeriac)

Chives

Cucumbers

Eggplant

Green beans

Kale

Lettuce (all varieties, including endive, iceberg, and romaine)

Parsnips

Potatoes (including red and white)

Radishes

Rutabaga

Summer squash (all varieties, including pattypan, yellow, and zucchini)

Spinach

Sweet potatoes (up to ½ cup per serving)

Swiss chard

Tomatoes

Turnips

Water chestnuts

Watercress

Shopping and Storage Tips

Of course, fresh is best when purchasing vegetables. Frozen would be your next best choice. Try to avoid canned vegetables, which tend to be higher in belly-bloating sodium. Choose brightly colored vegetables free of bruises. Baby carrots, prewashed and ready to eat, are a great choice. Look for baby greens such as baby spinach, baby bok choy, and baby kale, which are more tender and often a bit less bitter than the regular variety. Pick up some fresh herbs such as rosemary, thyme, and chives—these will provide flavor without troublesome FOD-MAPs. Remember, though, that some otherwise healthy vegetables, such as onions, asparagus, sugar snap peas, and cauliflower, are high in FODMAPs, so keep them out of your cart for now. (See Appendix B for a complete list of vegetables to avoid.)

Note that fresh and canned tomatoes are both allowed. Just be sure to choose brands that have no onions or garlic (both FODMAPs) and are low in sodium. Limit tomato paste to no more than 1 tablespoon per serving. Because it's concentrated, tomato paste has excess fructose that can bother your belly. Similarly, be careful with commercial tomato sauces, which often have added sugar, salt, or onions and garlic. Instead,

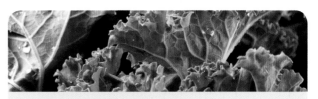

SPOTLIGHT ON *Kale*

Kale tops the list of modern-day superfoods, and for good reason. One cup of cooked kale has a mere 36 calories and 94 milligrams of calcium. Unlike many other leafy greens that contain oxalates that bind calcium in the greens, the calcium in kale is readily absorbed. Plus kale provides a nice dose of lutein and zeaxanthin, key nutrients known to lower the risk of developing macular degeneration, the leading cause of blindness in the elderly. Researchers are interested in indole-3-carbinol, prevalent in kale, for its cancer prevention and anti-inflammatory properties, which illustrates one more reason to enjoy this delicious leafy green.[1]

Kale is very versatile. Wilt it for a quick side dish, slice it finely for a yummy salad, or process it to turn it into a pesto or spread. Kale may even be blended in a smoothie if you want a green power drink. Kale comes in varieties such as curly, lacinato (also called dinosaur kale), and even reddish kale called redbor. Baby kale leaves, which are more tender than regular kale, make a wonderful salad. Still not sure how to cook with kale? Try Italian Tomato and Meatball Soup (page 115), Creamed Kale with Bacon and Hazelnuts (page 235), or Arroz con Pollo (page 184).

try making your own. Just chop up fresh tomatoes, add a little lemon juice, and simmer until it's at the consistency you like.

Most fresh produce should be refrigerated. Leafy greens and fresh herbs can be kept longer if you rinse and dry them and layer all of the leaves between sheets of paper towel. Stored this way in your crisper, leafy greens should last for up to a week. Root vegetables, such as potatoes and sweet potatoes, should be stored in a cool, dry, and dark area for up to 2 weeks for best freshness.

Cooking Tips

Frying your vegetables in a pro-inflammatory fat such as butter (rich in saturated fat) or corn oil (full of omega-6s) will negate most of the health benefits of your produce. Boiling your veggies will allow water-soluble vitamins, such as vitamin C and the B vitamins, to leach out and get lost in the water. So to maximize their nutrient content—and their flavor—steam or roast your veggies or serve them raw.

If you're used to having your vegetables covered in bread crumbs or smothered in sauce, you'll be pleasantly surprised to discover that fresh vegetables have so much flavor they hardly need any seasoning. But remember that tummy-soothing food doesn't have to be plain. Here are some belly-friendly ways to dress up your vegetables:

- Drizzle with a little sesame oil and a splash of reduced-sodium soy sauce (choose a gluten-free brand of soy sauce if you have gluten issues).

- Sprinkle with chopped fresh dill and a splash of lemon juice.

- Drizzle with balsamic vinegar or one of the Basic Salad Dressings on page 54.

- Sauté in Roasted Garlic Oil (see page 54) and garnish with fresh chives.

Some of the Belly Buddy veggies may be new to you, but don't be afraid of these versatile nutrient powerhouses. Isn't it time you discovered your roots? Turnips, rutabaga, and sweet potatoes make a wonderful side dish when roasted with a bit of olive oil, sea salt, and fresh thyme leaves. Haven't tried parsnips? Slice some up—they make a nice, spicy addition to a hearty stew.

Belly Buddy #2: Balanced-Fructose Fruits

All fruits contain fructose, which is often poorly digested and rapidly fermentable, thus making it a FODMAP. On the 21-Day Tummy plan, Kate and I have included fruits with a balanced glucose-to-fructose ratio, which are often digested more easily. That's because glucose helps your body absorb the fructose.

BALANCED-FRUCTOSE FRUITS

Bananas	Limes
Blueberries	Oranges
Cantaloupe	Papaya
Cranberries	Passion fruit
Grapes	Pineapple
Honeydew	Raspberries
Kiwis	Star fruit
Lemons	Strawberries

Shopping and Storage Tips

Fresh, seasonal fruits are your best choice for flavor and good nutrition. But frozen fruits can be more economical in cooler climates or seasons. Just be sure to choose those with no added sugar or preservatives, which can add calories and may even bother your stomach. Purchasing a few frozen bags

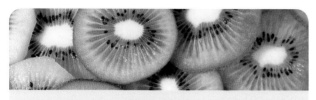

SPOTLIGHT ON *Kiwi*

Kiwi, a small tropical fruit with fuzzy skin, is a powerhouse of nutrition. In addition to vitamin C and potassium, kiwis stimulate the production of gut mucin, which helps maintain a healthy barrier in the intestine. That barrier is the frontline defense for keeping bad pathogens out of our body.[2] Kiwis also help our body digest protein in the stomach. For this reason, kiwi may be a great digestive aid.[3] We combine kiwi with protein in a slew of recipes, but my favorite is the Margarita Shrimp Salad (page 202). Additionally, the Kiwi and Orange Salad (page 220) recipe makes a nice accompaniment to grilled chicken, fish, or beef.

Just remember, kiwi is rich in enzymes that break down protein, so it can make ready-to-eat protein-rich foods (chicken, fish, Greek yogurt) turn mushy or curdle if added to the recipes ahead of time. For this reason, don't add kiwi to your smoothie unless you plan on drinking it right away, and don't add kiwi to cooked protein-rich dishes until right before you eat them! But, if you want to add kiwi to tougher cuts of raw meat, its protein-degrading enzyme, actinidin, will be a natural meat tenderizer.

of your favorite Belly Buddy fruits will simplify making your Belly Soother Smoothies: Just add frozen fruit (no dicing or peeling) and whirl up your favorite recipe.

Tropical fruits in particular, such as papaya or pineapple, may not be available fresh year-round. Look for frozen papaya or pineapple chunks in the freezer section or choose canned pineapple chunks (canned in their own juice, not in heavy syrup). Asian or other ethnic markets may also be good places to find exotic fruits, including the star fruit, a yellow-ridged oblong fruit that tastes a bit like a cross between an apple and pear and that slices into the cutest little starfish shape.

Most fruits are best stored in the refrigerator, and the majority last about 3 to 5 days. Bananas ripen best at room temperature. And no need to toss your overripe bananas. I like to freeze them for future use in my Belly Soother Smoothies! Simply peel, place in individual plastic storage bags, and toss in the freezer.

Cooking Tips

Most of your Belly Buddy fruits are best enjoyed fresh and raw as snacks or to round out a meal. But you'll also find fruits in some unexpected places. Grapes add a burst of sweetness to

Toasted Oat Muesli with Peanuts and Grapes (page 96); pineapples lend a tangy tenderness to Seared Pork Chops with Pineapple Sauce (page 134); and berries take center stage in several of our delectable desserts, from Raspberry Fool (page 266) to Berry-Studded Rice Pudding (page 272) and Blueberry Shortcakes (page 281).

Belly Buddy #3: Low FODMAP, High-Fiber Grains

It's axiomatic that fiber is good for your digestion and that grains, especially whole grains, are the best sources of fiber. That's true. But almost all grains are carb-dense (though whole grains are less carb-dense than refined grains), and many of the most popular grains today, including wheat, barley, and rye, are also full of FODMAPs. There are a handful of grains, though, that are rich in fiber, relatively carb-light, and low in the rapidly fermentable carbs that create gas and bloating. As an added bonus, they are also a good source of anti-inflammatory magnesium. You'll find these lighter grains in the later phases of the diet.

LOW-FODMAP GRAINS

Brown rice	Oats (whole)
Buckwheat	Polenta
Cornmeal	Quinoa
Corn tortillas	Rice bran
Oat bran	

Shopping and Storage Tips

No need to go to a specialty store to purchase these Belly Buddy grains. Most can be found on your everyday grocer's shelves. Check out the rice or bulk-food section for grains such as buckwheat, quinoa, polenta, and brown rice. Oats, oat bran,

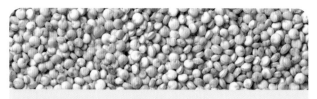

SPOTLIGHT ON *Quinoa*

Quinoa (pronounced "KEEN-wah") is considered an ancient grain native to the Andes, but it is really more of a seed than a cereal grain. Quinoa is naturally gluten free and protein rich and is loaded with vitamins and minerals, including thiamin, vitamin B6, iron, folate, zinc, potassium, and selenium, as well as the anti-inflammatory mineral magnesium.

Quinoa comes in a variety of colors: white, brown, black, and red. Red quinoa is a bit sweeter than the white variety. Brown, red, and black are a bit nuttier, while white cooks up to a smoother and creamier consistency.

Before cooking, rinse quinoa several times in cold water to remove the outer coating of bitter-tasting saponins. Kate finds that her patients are less likely to experience GI symptoms when they rinse quinoa, perhaps because saponins can impede protein digestion. Some brands of quinoa, such as Bob's Red Mill and Ancient Harvest, are pre-rinsed, so look for those to save time.

Quinoa is a quick-cooking grain: Boil it in water, then simmer and cover, and let the seeds cook for 10 to 15 minutes. You know quinoa is done cooking when the germ is partially detached and looks like a spiral coming off the seed. Enjoy quinoa in recipes where you would normally use rice or pasta.

and rice bran are typically found in the cereal section. When choosing oats for your oatmeal, select old-fashioned or rolled, with no added sugars, salt, or preservatives.

Cornmeal and polenta (which is made from ground cornmeal) are lower in FODMAPs compared to fresh sweet corn, which contains GOS and sorbitol. Limit fresh corn to just half a cob or about half a cup. Corn tortillas generally don't seem to cause digestive symptoms, so they can be a good option; stick with soft tortillas, though, not the hard ones, which are usually fried in pro-inflammatory oils. And avoid popcorn, which is carb-dense and sometimes contains trans fats.

If your grocery store has one, check out the gluten-free section. Here you'll find alternatives to refined wheat pasta, such as brown rice pasta, corn-quinoa pasta, or buckwheat noodles. (You may also find buckwheat noodles labeled as "soba," their Japanese name, in the Asian section. But check the ingredients labels carefully; many soba noodles are actually buckwheat–wheat flour blends.) Not only are these delicious gluten-free pasta substitutes, they are lower in FODMAPs.

Your Belly Buddy grains are best stored in an airtight container in your pantry. If you don't intend to use up your grains within a month or so, you can store them in the freezer. This prevents the unsaturated fats in the germ of whole grains from going rancid, extending their shelf life.

Cooking Tips

No doubt you're familiar with oatmeal, but did you know that oat bran can also make a delicious hot cereal? The outer portion of the oat grain, oat bran is rich in soluble fiber and has been shown to lower blood cholesterol.[4] I love this carb-light, magnesium-rich grain cooked up and topped with blueberries, cinnamon, and pecans. Or try it as a crunchy topping in the Breakfast Fruit Salad (page 99). This delightful breakfast treat just might start your love affair with oat bran! Oat bran can also be used in place of bread crumbs in savory dishes such as Veggie Patties with Chipotle Mayo (page 160) and Crispy-Topped Broiled Tomatoes (page 243).

> The delightful Breakfast Fruit Salad just might start your love affair with oat bran!

Buckwheat, despite its name, is not related to wheat. Roasted kernels of buckwheat are called kasha and are commonly used in Eastern European cuisines as a hot cereal or as a side dish, like our Sunny Kasha (page 260).

Belly Buddy #4: Nuts and Nut Butters

Nuts and nut butters are not only filling and tasty, but also a great source of healthy fats (more on these later) and magnesium. Walnuts are a source of heart-healthy omega-3 fats, the only nut that has that honor. But our top choice in this section is good old-fashioned peanuts because they are one

FOODS IN FOCUS: TUMMY TWISTERS OR TUMMY TAMERS?

Sometimes old wives' tales have us erroneously thinking certain foods are ideal to calm our belly when they may in fact get our gut in a rut. **White toast** and **applesauce,** for instance, are often prescribed to cure the runs. But both are rich in FOD-MAPs, so they may actually make diarrhea worse.

Berries are touted as antioxidant and fiber-rich nutritional superstars, but not all berries are gentle on your tummy. Strawberries, raspberries, and blueberries are yummy Tummy Tamers, but blackberries are a Tummy Twister loaded with naturally occuring sorbitol, a FODMAP.

All nuts have belly-soothing healthy fats, but some, such as pistachios and cashews, are also rich in fructans and GOS, both FODMAPs, so they are not allowed on the 21-Day Tummy plan. Almonds and hazelnuts are a little high in FODMAPs, so stick to 10 nuts or about 1 tablespoon of nut butter per serving.

Conversely, while many people think **acidic foods** cause acid reflux, research shows that this is not the case. Acid reflux occurs when stomach acid rises up through the lower esophageal sphincter (LES). Protein-rich foods increase LES pressure (a good thing), while fat lowers LES pressure and contributes to acid reflux. Acidic foods do not alter LES pressure, which is why we have included fresh tomatoes and oranges in the 21-Day Tummy diet. But if you have untreated acid reflux that has irritated your esophagus, acidic foods act like salt in the wound; in this case, you might want to try milder fruits.

Common cabbage also has a reputation as a Tummy Twister that is undeserved. While savoy and napa cabbage are relatively high in FODMAPs, regular green cabbage is actually low-calorie, fiber-rich, and filling Tummy Tamers.

Soybeans (dried and edamame) and **soy flour** contain tummy-twisting GOS and fructans. But fermented soybeans (tempeh) and firm tofu have the majority of the FODMAPs removed in processing, making them excellent tummy-taming protein sources, especially for vegetarians and vegans.

of our best sources of anti-inflammatory magnesium: Two tablespoons of peanut butter or 30 peanuts contain 49 milligrams. Since nuts are high in calories, limit yourself to just a handful with each serving. You'll want to be especially careful with almonds and hazelnuts, which are a little higher in FOD-MAPs (have no more than 10 nuts per serving), and for the duration of the 21-Day Tummy plan, we suggest you avoid cashews and pistachios, which have large amounts of fructans and GOS. Peanuts, walnuts, and pecans are lowest in FODMAPs.

NUTS AND NUT BUTTERS

Almonds (up to 10 nuts or 1 tablespoon nut butter per serving)
Hazelnuts (up to 10 nuts or 1 tablespoon nut butter per serving)
Macadamia nuts
Peanuts
Pecans
Pine nuts
Walnuts

(continued on page 36)

Sabrina Ng, Age 31

**LOST 6 POUNDS and
1¾ BELLY INCHES IN 21 DAYS!**

Sabrina Ng works in ad sales, so entertaining clients is a big part of her life. In addition, this single gal has an active social life, frequently enjoying dinners with family and drinks with the girls. All of this wining and dining, of course, took a toll on her waistline. In addition, she suffered from regular abdominal cramps, gas, bloating, diarrhea, nausea, and acid reflux.

For Sabrina, doing her belly good meant rethinking what it meant to have a good time. It also meant being open to trying new foods and new ways of cooking, as well as learning what appropriate portions were for some of her old favorites. Having never stuck to a strict meal plan before, she found the 21-day

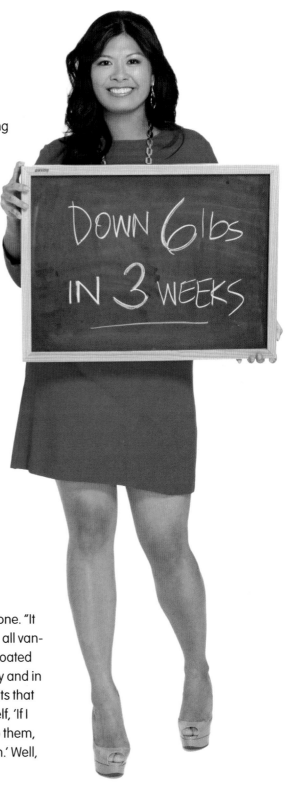

A Social Butterfly Trims Her Tummy

plan a challenge at first, but a worthwhile one. "It works!" she exclaims. Her digestive issues all vanished and, she says, "I feel so much less bloated after this diet. I love the changes in my belly and in how my clothes fit. There was a pair of pants that I bought before this diet, and I said to myself, 'If I lose 5 pounds in the next 3 weeks, I'll keep them, and if I can't lose the weight, I'll return them.' Well, I'm keeping those pants!"

(continued from page 34)
Shopping and Storage Tips

Nuts should be plump and uniform in size and color. Both roasted and raw nuts are healthy choices, but if you choose roasted nuts, avoid varieties that contain other FODMAP ingredients such as onion powder or belly-bloating added salt (they are also often contaminated with gluten). Nuts should be stored in an airtight container in the refrigerator and should stay fresh for up to 6 months.

When purchasing nut butters, it is best to use all-natural nut butters made from the nuts alone. These preservative-free nut butters should be stored in your refrigerator for longest shelf life and consumed by the use-by date noted on the jar. Many traditional peanut butters add partially hydrogenated fats, also known as pro-inflammatory trans fats, so be sure to check the labels.

Cooking Tips

Adding a small amount of nuts or nut butters to meals adds an anti-inflammation boost due to monounsaturated fats and magnesium. But don't get carried away: Nuts and nut butters should be used sparingly as they are rich in calories. Just half a cup of almonds contains more than 400 calories—more than most of the meals in this plan!

Luckily, it doesn't take a lot of nuts to add the satisfying flavor and texture you crave. A handful of nuts, paired with a banana or carrot sticks, makes a quick and easy snack. Ground hazelnuts make the perfect stuffing for Hazelnut-Stuffed Pork Chops (page 132); sliced almonds add a nice crunch to the Crisp Green Salad with Nuts in a Ginger Dressing (page 217); and rich peanut butter gets baked into the flourless Chocolate-Covered Peanut Butter Cookies (page 276). You will find nuts lightly dispersed among the recipes and the 21-Day Tummy plan, just enough to provide all the health benefits without tipping the calories out of control.

Belly Buddy #5: Seeds

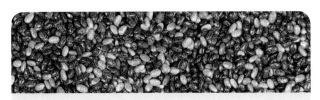

Seeds are a great source of fiber and healthy fats. Sprinkle 1 tablespoon of chia seeds on some Greek yogurt or your salad, and you have a nutritious 5-gram fiber boost. Chia and flaxseeds, known as valuable sources of soluble fiber (which helps lower your bad cholesterol and aid digestion) and omega-3 fats (which fights inflammation), are great for your ticker and your tummy. Pumpkin seeds, a magnesium powerhouse, provide almost 200 milligrams in a mere quarter cup, or almost two-thirds of an adult woman's needs per day.

SPOTLIGHT ON *Chia*

Yes, what used to embellish sculpture heads or animal models and grow into grasslike stems is now prepared for human consumption. Chia seeds are low-FODMAP, high-fiber seeds—and one tablespoon contains as much calcium as a quarter cup of milk! Unlike flaxseeds, chia seeds do not need to be ground prior to eating them and can be stored at room temperature until the best-by date on the package.

Enjoy chia on top of your morning oats, blended into a smoothie, sprinkled on your salad, mixed into one of our delicious recipes, such as the Quinoa and Oat Bran Cereal (page 93), or as a topping on the Crispy-Topped Broiled Tomatoes (page 243). Chia has it all: cholesterol-lowering soluble fiber, anti-inflammation magnesium, and bone-strengthening calcium. Chia is getting a bit more mainstream these days, so you should be able to purchase some at your local grocery store. Look in the baking section or perhaps the bulk food aisle.

SEEDS

Chia seeds   Sesame seeds
Flaxseeds   Sunflower seeds
Pumpkin seeds

Shopping and Storage Tips

Be sure to buy unsalted seeds with no seasoning added, especially if you have celiac disease, as they may be contaminated with gluten in the processing.

Chia seeds and flaxseeds may be found more readily in health food stores, but more conventional stores are now carrying them, too. Flaxseeds should be ground prior to consumption to allow your body to adequately benefit and absorb all of their nutrients. You can do this yourself by grinding them in a coffee mill, or purchase flaxseed meal and the extra work is done for you! If you purchase flaxseed meal, store it in the refrigerator in an airtight container until the best-by date on the package.

Pumpkin seeds can be purchased in their shell or hulled. Hulled pumpkin seeds are called pepitas. I like pepitas as they are easy to pop in my smoothie or top on my oats. They are my personal favorite magnesium booster!

Cooking Tips

Toasting seeds such as sesame, pumpkin, or chia in a skillet on your stovetop will maximize their flavor. Just cook them in a small skillet over medium-low heat, stirring constantly, until lightly browned. (Be especially careful with pumpkin and sesame seeds, which tend to pop.) Small amounts of sesame seeds are allowed on the 21-Day Tummy plan, but sesame seed paste (tahini) has been found to be high in FODMAPs, so avoid it while following the plan.

> I like pepitas as they are easy to pop in my smoothie or top on my oats. They are my personal favorite magnesium booster!

You can also roast whole pumpkin seeds. Just spread them on an oiled cookie sheet, sprinkle with salt, and bake in a preheated oven at 325 degrees Fahrenheit until they're golden brown. (This can take anywhere from 5 to 20 minutes, depending on how big the seeds are.) You may want to flip them halfway through the cook time. You can eat the shells, which add fiber, or crack them open to get to the meaty seed inside.

Belly Buddy #6: Healthy Fats

Fat has gotten a bad rap, touted as the evil villain in the war on obesity and heart disease. But not all fats are created equal. In fact, omega-3 fats, found primarily in fish, and monounsaturated fats (MUFAs), found primary in olive oil and nuts, actively fight inflammation.

It's best to get healthy fats from a mix of foods (some fish, some oils, some olives or avocados) because each offers other important nutrients and a nice blend of omega-3s and MUFAs.

HEALTHY FATS

Omega-3 Fatty Acids

Herring
Mackerel
Salmon
Sardines
Tuna

Flaxseeds and flaxseed oil
Rapeseed (canola) oil
Soybean oil
Walnuts and walnut oil

MUFAs

Avocados (up to ⅛ avocado or ¼ cup diced avocado per serving)

Dark chocolate
Nuts and seeds
Olives and olive oil
Sesame oil

Shopping and Storage Tips

Fish: When purchasing fish, select markets that are busy with good turnover, which often translates to fresher fish for you. Be sure the fish is covered with ice both top and bottom. When purchasing fish fillets, choose those with moist, resilient skin and avoid those with any discoloration or gaps in the flesh. Smell is a good indicator of freshness. If it smells briny, bring it home; if it has a "fishy" odor, leave it at the store! Frozen fish is another healthy option. Avoid fish that shows signs of freezer burn, which appears like a white and crusty texture on the flesh, indicating the fish has been frozen incorrectly or for too long. Store fish, wrapped in plastic wrap, in the coldest part of your refrigerator. Use within 24 hours of purchase or freeze for up to 6 months.

Olive, seed, and nut oils: Choose olive oil that is minimally processed, such as extra-virgin or cold-pressed olive oil. When purchasing oils such as sesame to infuse an Asian flavor or olive oil for salad dressing, choose small bottles (large containers of oils are exposed to more oxygen every time you open the bottle; this contributes to the oil's rancidity). Sesame oil, generally speaking, will be found in the Asian section of the grocery store near the soy sauce. Other nut-based oils will be found near the salad dressings. Choose pure oils over oil blends, and store them in a cool, dark place or in the refrigerator. Oils will retain flavor and freshness for about 6 months.

> Mixing up some easy, belly-friendly marinades and sauces can be a tasty way to flavor your fish.

Olives: Olives, which are pickled in brine or dry-cured, are often high in sodium. Look for lower sodium olives, which are often available. Bottled or canned olives, once opened, should be stored in the refrigerator and used within 2 months.

Avocados: If you are picking up an avocado to use right away, look for one that yields to gentle pressure. If you plan to use it later in the week, select a firmer one. Store your avocado at room temperature for proper ripening. Once cut, an avocado will turn brown, so add a bit of lemon or lime juice to maintain the green color.

Chocolate: Semisweet or dark chocolate is the preferred chocolate on the 21-Day Tummy plan as it is richest in antioxidants and lower in lactose. Avoid milk chocolate, which is a source of lactose. If you can see the chocolate under the packaging, look for a smooth and shiny surface. Store chocolate tightly sealed and in a cool dry place for up to 1 year.

Cooking Tips

Fish: Grill, bake, braise, broil, or even microwave your fish. Yes, microwaving an individual 6-ounce serving of a salmon fillet should take less than 4 minutes. Now that's fast food! Of course, avoid fried fish, which is difficult on your digestive health not to mention damaging to your waistline. Mixing up some easy, belly-friendly marinades and sauces can be a tasty way to flavor your fish. I like to mix freshly squeezed lemon juice, a drizzle of Roasted Garlic Oil (page 54), and a teaspoon of Dijon mustard and then brush it on raw shrimp, swordfish, or salmon; grill, bake, or broil the fish, then garnish with chopped fresh basil. Or, for a quick Asian dressing, try a 2:1 blend of soy sauce and sesame oil, mixed with a few black sesame seeds and then brushed onto your salmon or tuna steak before grilling or broiling it.

Olive, seed, and nut oils: Drizzle a tablespoon over salad greens. Brush a little oil on fish or veggies to keep them moist prior to grilling, baking, or broiling. I love a drizzle of sesame oil to season a delicious stir-fry or sautéed green beans. Peanut oil provides a nutty flavor to my Asian stir-fries.

Olives: Add a few olives to your salad for a healthy dose of anti-inflammatory fats. Chop some up and add to ground meat to kick up the flavor of a lean burger or meat loaf. Or blend olives into a tapenade to enjoy on a brown rice cracker or red pepper strip.

Avocados: Keep portions small (no more than ⅛ avocado per serving) to keep your FODMAP and calorie intake in the safe zone. Garnish your favorite Mexican-inspired dishes with a handful of diced avocado. Top scrambled eggs with a few slices plus chopped fresh cilantro and diced tomatoes. Avocado also pairs well with tuna or chicken.

Chocolate: Chocolate should be savored in small amounts. Perhaps top your Greek yogurt with a tablespoon of semisweet chocolate chips. Or try my favorite on-the-go snack: a sliced banana, a small dollop of almond butter, and a few chocolate chips. Mmmm.

Belly Buddy #7: Lean Protein

Want to feel more satisfied after eating a meal? Then be sure to add some lean protein. Because protein lessens our temptation to snack, protein-rich diets are associated with greater weight loss.

Fish is one of the best protein sources as it is low in calories and rich in tummy-friendly omega-3 fats—particularly fatty fish such as salmon, tuna, and swordfish. Poultry, especially boneless and skinless white meat chicken or turkey, is also a light and lean choice. Select cuts of pork can be low in fat, too, especially center-cut pork loin chops or tenderloin. Beef tends to be the highest in fat, but lean sources such as London broil and flank steak can be enjoyed once a week. And if you want to go meatless, try tofu or tempeh, which, due to processing, are lower in FODMAPs compared to other soybean products and thus easier on digestion. Other commonly consumed plant-based protein such as beans offer many hardworking nutrients, such as cholesterol-lowering fiber and anti-inflammatory magnesium. But they can be tough on the gut due to their high GOS content, which can make you gassy!

LEAN PROTEIN

Eggs

Fish (especially those high in omega-3 fats, listed above)

Lean cuts of beef (such as flank steak, London broil, and tenderloin; 95% lean ground beef)

Lean cuts of pork (such as center-cut loin chops and tenderloin)

Poultry (such as boneless, skinless chicken and turkey breast)

Seafood (including shellfish such as shrimp, crabs, lobster, mussels, oysters, and clams)

Tempeh

Tofu

Shopping and Storage Tips

Eggs: Choose eggs that are enhanced with omega-3s for anti-inflammation benefits. Eggs labeled with the USDA organic program labels means that the eggs were laid by uncaged hens that are fed an organic diet free of conventional pesticides or fertilizers. The nutrient content of organic versus conventional eggs does not differ, but limiting pesticide and fertilizer exposure might be a good thing! Store eggs in the refrigerator for up to 3 weeks or use by the best-by date on the package.

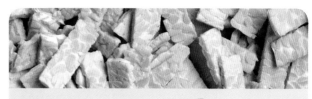

SPOTLIGHT ON *Tempeh*

Tempeh is a vegan protein source made from cooked and fermented soybeans. Unlike whole unfermented soybeans, such as edamame, which contain GOS, tempeh is low in FODMAPs. The fermentation process lowers the GOS levels to tolerable amounts. A 4-ounce serving of tempeh provides 12 grams of fiber and 22 grams of protein, and does not contain any cholesterol, which is true of all plant foods. Avoid tempeh products with barley, onions, or other potential Belly Bully ingredients. I like to brush tempeh with a mixture of soy sauce and sesame oil and grill it, slice it, and serve it over a stir-fry or salad.

Fish and seafood: As with the omega-3-rich fish described on page 39, avoid fish or seafood with any discoloration or gaps and any that smell fishy. Store fish, wrapped in plastic wrap, and shellfish and other seafood in a shallow pan on a bed of ice in the coldest part of your refrigerator. Use within 24 hours of purchase or freeze for up to 6 months.

Beef, pork, and poultry: Stick to the lean cuts indicated in this section to keep your calorie and saturated fat intake to a minimum. In particular, limit your consumption of beef and other red meat to once a week. When shopping for meat, steer clear of any cuts with visible marbled fat, and trim as much external fat as you can from the meat before cooking. Keep meat in its original packaging, and safely freeze for 6 to 12 months. Or you can refrigerate poultry and ground meat for 2 days, beef and pork up to 5 days. Avoid any prepared meats such as meatballs or sausages, which often have extra fat, salt, bread crumbs, garlic, onion, or other tummy-troubling ingredients added.

Tofu and tempeh: These can sometimes be found in the produce section, sometimes in the Asian food section of the grocery store. As these hearty vegan proteins have become more popular, more flavors and varieties have appeared on shelves. But basic is best here—your top choices will be unflavored extra-firm tofu and unflavored tempeh, which will have the fewest FODMAPs. Tempeh and tofu should be stored in the refrigerator and used by the best-by date on the package.

Cooking Tips

Eggs: Eggs are a terrific source of protein and easy on the wallet. They make for a hearty breakfast but can protein-pack lunch or dinner, too! Simply cook a beaten egg into your favorite rice or noodle dish, or top your mixed green salad with a hard-cooked egg to boost your tummy-taming protein.

Fish and seafood: Fish is great grilled, baked, braised, broiled, or even microwaved. Shrimp and scallops cook up in a flash stir-fried in a skillet or simply seared. They are wonderful grilled, too. Lobster and clams are best steamed or boiled.

Beef, pork, and poultry: Enjoy these meats baked, grilled, broiled, or sautéed for a healthy and tasty meal. Of course, breading and/or frying should be avoided due to the pro-inflammatory fats used in frying and the FODMAP ingredients (wheat, onion, garlic) often present in the breading.

Tofu and tempeh: These soy-based proteins make great additions to a veggie stir-fry. Marinate tofu or tempeh in a soy sauce–based dressing, slice it up, and add to a stir-fry. Tempeh's firmer texture makes it easy to grill, too.

These simple combinations add some flavor and pizzazz to your protein dish. Try them on different types of protein.

- Place fresh dill and sliced lemon directly on your meat, fish, or poultry prior to baking.

- Sprinkle ground thyme and black pepper generously over meat, fish, or poultry, and bake or grill.

- Rub Jerk Rub (page 53) over chicken, beef, tofu, tempeh, or fish, and bake or grill.

- Blend 1 teaspoon Dijon mustard and 2 teaspoons maple syrup (can double or triple recipe as needed). Brush over chicken, beef, or pork, and bake or grill.

- Mix 2 tablespoons nonfat plain Greek yogurt with ¼ teaspoon onion-free curry powder and a dash of salt and pepper. Brush over chicken, beef, pork, tempeh, or tofu and bake.

- Mix 2 tablespoons reduced-sodium tamari (soy sauce), 1 tablespoon water, 1 teaspoon sesame oil, and 1 teaspoon sesame seeds. Marinate tofu, tempeh, chicken, pork, fish, or beef in this mixture for about 30 minutes (recipe can be doubled or tripled as needed). Remove from the marinade, then stir-fry, grill, or bake.

PROBIOTICS AND PREBIOTICS

Probiotics are microbes (usually bacteria or yeast) that provide a healthy benefit to the body. Prebiotics are fibers that promote the growth of probiotics. Probiotic and prebiotic supplements can be found in yogurts, cereals, and even chocolate bars, as well as in pill form. The explosion of probiotics and prebiotics in the marketplace have all been prompted by the expanding research that shows that probiotic bacteria help keep our gut bacteria in balance. But since each of us has our own gut bacterial "fingerprint," a supplement that helps me may not help you.

In addition, one of the most common prebiotics—inulin, sometimes listed on labels as chicory root extract or FOS—is a FODMAP and thus may trigger digestive woes for those sensitive to them.

For these reasons, Kate and I encourage you to get your probiotics from food, rather than from supplements. (Also, we want to make sure the plan's healing foods are doing their work. If you are already taking probiotics, though, and find them helpful, by all means continue using them.) Greek yogurt is a great source of naturally occurring probiotics. Many fermented foods, such as sauerkraut and kefir, have probiotic microbes, too.

Belly Buddy #8: Greek Yogurt

Greek yogurt is the latest craze to hit the grocer's dairy aisle. It has twice the protein content of regular yogurt and less lactose, a plus for anyone who might be lactose-intolerant. This is because most of the milk sugar, lactose, is drained out when making this thicker-style yogurt. It is also a source of probiotics, healthy bacteria that may help settle your stomach. We included Greek yogurt throughout the plan as an easy grab-and-go snack and as the protein-rich base in our Belly Soother Smoothie.

Shopping and Storage Tips

Choose nonfat plain Greek yogurt to avoid inflammatory saturated fat and save on calories. Avoid flavorings, which may include FODMAP-full inulin (chicory root extract) and/or carb-dense sugar. Always check expiration dates and store in your refrigerator up until that date. You can also freeze the yogurt: Fill ice cube trays or small freezer bags about two-thirds full with yogurt, which you can easily portion out to use in your smoothies or other desserts.

If you are extra sensitive to lactose, you can sub in lactose-free yogurt in place of Greek yogurt.

Cooking Tips

Greek yogurt makes a great substitute for lactose-rich sour cream in your favorite dip recipes or as a topping on baked potatoes and baked goods. Greek yogurt also makes a delightfully creamy dressing: Just combine it with lemon juice, maple syrup, and a touch of oil. Drizzle it on salads, as in the Chicken Ambrosia (page 189), or use it as a marinade for chicken, fish, or tofu. And, of course, plain Greek yogurt all by itself makes a quick and filling breakfast, snack, or dessert. Top it with fresh fruit, vanilla extract, chia seeds, and maybe a drizzle of maple syrup for a scrumptious, stomach-soothing flavor boost.

Belly Buddy #9: Coconut Milk

In addition to its delicious flavor, coconut milk is a source of medium-chain triglycerides (MCTs), a type of fat with an unusual chemical structure that allows it to be digested more easily. Most fats require bile or digestive enzymes to be digested properly, but MCTs are absorbed intact and taken to the liver where they are used directly for energy. And, while the effect appears to be slight, researchers from McGill University in Montreal Canada found that a diet rich in MCTs may even increase calorie burning.[5] In addition to coconut milk, coconut oil is also rich in MCTs.

Shopping and Storage Tips

Coconut milk can be purchased in boxes or cans. Boxed varieties tend to have less calories and fat (23 calories and 2.3 grams of fat per half cup) but sometimes have more additives, so be sure to choose unsweetened versions and avoid products with added sugar or inulin. Unsweetened canned light coconut milk is another great option, although it has a higher calorie and fat content (70 calories and 6 grams of fat per half cup serving).

Unopened coconut milk is shelf stable, but once you've opened a box or can, either refrigerate for one week or freeze it. Pour the coconut milk into ice cube trays that will be easy to pop out and use in your Belly Soother Smoothies.

Cooking Tips

Canned coconut milk is creamier than the boxed variety and adds a terrific velvety texture to many of the recipes in this cookbook, from your Belly Soother Smoothies (page 85) to Tofu Coconut Curry (page 205). Choose the lower-calorie boxed coconut milk when you're looking for a refreshing lactose-free milk substitute to drink.

Belly Buddy #10: Ginger

Ginger has long been used as a remedy to quell nausea. What really put ginger on the Belly Buddy list, though, is its ability to help the stomach contract and empty its contents, aiding digestion.[6] Ginger is also well known for its anti-inflammatory properties, including its ability to reduce the onset and progression of rheumatoid arthritis in an animal study.[7] By now, you know that beating inflammation is key to keeping your tummy calm and trim. Moreover, we love the flavor ginger infuses in so many of the recipes in the *21-Day Tummy Diet Cookbook*.

Shopping and Storage Tips

When buying fresh ginger, look for a root that is plump and has unblemished skin. Jarred minced ginger is another option—it is often found in the Asian section of your grocery store. Pickled ginger is another tasty way to enjoy this Belly Buddy, but avoid products with added sorbitol, a source of FODMAPs. Candied ginger tastes delicious, and you could make your own with maple syrup in the oven, but avoid the many carb-dense commercial brands with copious amounts of added sugar.

> Ginger is well-known for its anti-inflammatory properties. Beating inflammation is key to keeping your tummy calm and trim.

Store fresh ginger in a sealed plastic bag (all air removed) in the refrigerator for up to 2 weeks, or store in the freezer for up to 2 months. You can also purchase dried ginger powder in the spice section of your grocery store.

Cooking Tips

Just a teaspoonful of grated ginger can add a little kick to your Belly Soother Smoothie or to hot oatmeal. And, of course, sliced ginger is a delicious addition to Asian-inspired stir-fry recipes, such as our Shrimp Stir-Fry (page 203). If you're substituting dried ginger powder for grated fresh ginger, use only about one-third the amount, as the dried variety is a concentrated source of this herb.

Belly Buddy #11: Turmeric

Ground turmeric (pronounced "TER-muh-rihk") is a staple in Indian and Middle Eastern cooking. Also known as Indian saffron, it is an earthy-tasting spice that gives curry its golden color. Curcumin, the active ingredient in turmeric, is well known for its potential cancer-preventing benefits, particularly colon and breast cancer. A recent study found that curcurmin helped change pro-inflammatory reactions to anti-inflammatory effects in individuals with inflammatory colitis and reduced their rate of relapse.[8]

RECOMMENDED BRANDS

Many spices and sauces, among other foods, may contain trace amounts of gluten. While most people with gluten intolerance can consume these without symptoms, for those with celiac disease these traces of gluten can be toxic! To be safe, we suggest that you look for brands known to be gluten free. Here are a few suggestions of gluten-free products to look for. Except where noted, these brands are also free of garlic and onions.

- Chobani nonfat plain Greek yogurt
- Fage nonfat plain Greek yogurt
- Laughing Cow Light Creamy Swiss spreadable cheese
- ReNew Life Ultimate ChiaLife
- Bob's Red Mill Gluten Free Oat Bran
- McCormick Chili Powder (contains onion)
- McCormick Chipotle Chile Pepper
- Spice Appeal Chili Powder
- Spice Appeal Curry Powder
- Pacific Organic Free Range Low Sodium Chicken Broth (contains onion)
- Lea & Perrins Worcestershire Sauce (contains onion)
- San-J Tamari Gluten-Free Soy Sauce
- Maille mustard
- Hunt's plain canned tomatoes
- Muir Glen fire-roasted canned tomatoes

Finally, if you're looking for lactose-free yogurt, try Green Valley Organics.

Shopping and Storage Tips

Find turmeric in the spice section of your grocer's baking aisle. Turmeric is also a key ingredient in most curry powders. Look for onion- and garlic-free brands of curry powder.

Cooking Tips

In addition to Indian dishes like Tandoori-Style Baked Chicken (page 138) and Middle Eastern dishes like Middle Eastern Chicken Skillet Dinner (page 179), try turmeric as a substitute in recipes that call for saffron or ground mustard for a flavor and health boost.

Belly Buddy #12: Maple Syrup

We all know that sugar packs on the pounds, but did you know that it also fuels inflammation? Granulated (table) sugar has 99.98 grams of carbohydrate per 100 grams. That's about as carb-dense as you can get—and the more carb-dense the food, the more likely it is to cause inflammation.

What about other common sweeteners? High-fructose corn syrup (HFCS) is so called because it has more fructose than glucose, making it a FODMAP. It's also high on the carb density scale, with 76 grams of carbohydrate per 100 grams. Stay clear of HFCS as it's linked with fatty liver, obesity, and digestive woes such as gas and bloating. Agave nectar is also a source of excess fructose and was a definite digestive trigger for me. Good-bye, agave! Stevia may be a natural sweetener, but most of the stevia products in the supermarket are a far cry from the plant as it's grown in nature, so I suggest you avoid those, too.

Sugar substitutes can be problematic for your tummy, as well. Sugar alcohols like sorbitol and mannitol are FOD-MAPs. Splenda (sucralose) may kill some of your healthy gut bacteria, while aspartame and saccharin may cause weight gain. You deserve real foods and so does your body. So Kate and I have pulled all artificial sugars off the table during the 21-Day Tummy plan.

Does that mean we have to give up on sweetness altogether?

(continued on page 52)

Jonathan Bigham, Age 43

LOST 7½ POUNDS and
1 BELLY INCH IN 21 DAYS!

Jonathan Bigham had always been trim and fit. But, he noted, "since I turned 40, I've been gaining weight only in the middle, and no matter how far I'd run or how many laps I'd do in the pool, nothing worked." Until the 21-Day Tummy plan, that is. After the plan, he crows, "I feel like I stand taller. I fit into pants that didn't fit 3 weeks ago. I've moved my belt notch back . . . and I'm less anxious about looking older than my age or having clothes that are too tight and uncomfortable."

He Kicked a 6-Bottle-a-Day Soda Habit

Jonathan was happily surprised at "how easy it was to actually be able to cook all my meals and that it didn't take a huge amount of time." He was even able to stick to the plan during his family vacation to Disney World. It helped that his energy levels skyrocketed on the plan. "Two weeks into the plan, and I've been waking up without the need for an alarm all week." He also found that vigorous activities such as his regular runs became easier, and his usual bouts of diarrhea and acid reflux completely disappeared. Plus, since he kicked his six-bottle-a-day diet soda habit, he's even saving money!

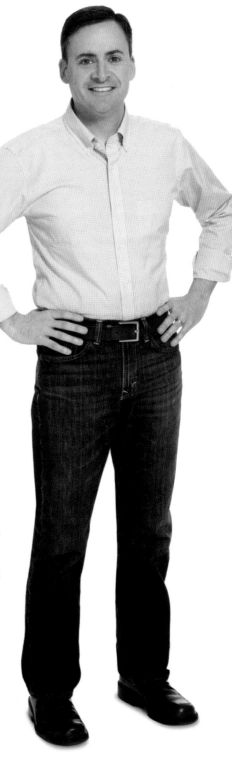

(continued from page 50)

While no sweeteners are truly carb-light, maple syrup comes in at a much lower density—67 grams per 100 grams—than other sweeteners. Plus, in a recent study, University of Rhode Island researchers discovered numerous phytochemicals in maple syrup that are powerful antioxidants, which may play as important a role in anti-inflammation as vitamin C.[9]

Shopping and Storage Tips

Purchase pure maple syrup, not its imposter, pancake syrup, which is often full of artificial ingredients including HFCS. Maple syrup comes in different grades, all of which are generally easy on your tummy: Grade A has three varieties (light, medium, and dark amber); grade B is darker and stronger. The darker the maple syrup, the more intense the flavor. Maple syrup can be stored at room temperature for about a year unopened; once opened, it must be refrigerated until its best-by date.

Cooking Tips

Maple syrup provides the needed sweetness to smoothies, desserts, and some salad dressings and marinades. You will find a hint of maple syrup added to recipes throughout the cookbook, including in the Spice-Rubbed Chicken with Grape Relish (page 143) and "Banana Splits" (page 271).

Spicing Up Your Life

Since many commercial spice blends and salad dressings are notorious for containing garlic and onion (both FODMAPs), here are a few recipes that provide all the flavor you want without troubling your tummy.

Taco Spice Blend

- 1 tablespoon chili powder (look for onion- and garlic-free brands such as Spice Appeal)
- 2 teaspoons ground cumin
- 2 teaspoons paprika
- ½ teaspoon fine sea salt

Mix and store in an airtight container for up to 12 months. Add 1 tablespoon to 1 pound of lean ground meat for Mexican flavor!

Curry Spice Blend

Note: Some blends are available without onion and garlic, such as Spice Appeal Curry Powder.

- 3 tablespoons paprika
- 2 teaspoons ground cumin
- ½ teaspoon ground fennel
- 2 teaspoons ground mustard
- 1 dash cayenne pepper
- 1 tablespoon ground coriander
- 1 tablespoon ground turmeric
- 1 teaspoon ground cardamom
- ½ teaspoon ground cinnamon
- ½ teaspoon ground cloves

Mix and store in an airtight container for up to 12 months. Enjoy this spice blend in rice-based dishes or in soups and stews.

Jerk Rub

- 1 tablespoon light brown sugar
- 1 tablespoon dried thyme, crumbled
- 1 teaspoon paprika
- 1½ teaspoons salt
- 1½ teaspoons ground allspice
- ½ teaspoon ground nutmeg
- ½ teaspoon ground cinnamon
- ½ teaspoon ground cloves
- ¼ teaspoon cayenne pepper, if tolerated

Mix and store in an airtight container for up to 12 months. Rub this tasty blend onto your fish, chicken, or pork before grilling or roasting.

Roasted Garlic Oil

12 cloves garlic, peeled and thickly sliced

¾ cup extra-virgin olive oil

Preheat the oven to 325°F. Submerge the garlic in the oil in a small baking dish. Cover tightly with foil and place on a baking sheet. Bake for 35 to 45 minutes, or until the garlic is just beginning to turn color. After it's cooled down, strain out and discard the garlic. Store the oil in a glass jar in the refrigerator for up to 10 days. Use this garlic-infused oil in place of plain olive oil anytime you want a little garlic flavor without the bothersome FODMAPs. You can also use this technique to infuse oil with onions and shallots.

Basic Salad Dressing

¾ cup olive oil

¼ cup red wine or rice vinegar

Salt and pepper, to taste

Dijon style: Whisk in 1 tablespoon Dijon mustard.

Dilly dressing: Whisk in 1 tablespoon chopped fresh dill.

Italian style: Sub in Roasted Garlic Oil (above) for the olive oil, and add ½ teaspoon dried basil and ½ teaspoon dried oregano.

Greek: Sub in Roasted Garlic Oil (above) for the olive oil, and add 1 tablespoon chopped fresh oregano and ¼ cup finely crumbled feta cheese.

Whisk the dressing ingredients to blend, store in a glass jar in the refrigerator, and use within 7 days.

THE 21-DAY TUMMY PANTRY

Keeping some 21-Day Tummy staples on hand will make it a snap to prepare belly-friendly meals in minutes. Here's a list of some items you may want to have at the ready:

Dry goods:
- Oat bran
- Rolled oats
- Quinoa
- Chia seeds
- Ground flaxseed
- Pumpkin seeds (pepitas)
- Almonds, whole and sliced
- All-natural peanut butter and/or almond butter
- Olive oil
- Sesame oil
- Soy sauce
- Balsamic vinegar

- Coconut milk: canned light or unsweetened box variety
- Turmeric
- Dried ginger powder
- Curry powder (without onion and garlic)

Refrigerated goods:
- Nonfat plain Greek yogurt
- Baby carrots
- Fresh ginger
- Maple syrup
- Dijon mustard (without onion and garlic)

- Lemons
- Bananas

Freezer staples:
- Frozen blueberries and strawberries
- Frozen veggies such as kale, spinach, green beans, and carrots
- Frozen shrimp, fish fillets, boneless skinless poultry, pork tenderloin, and flank steak

***

Don't be afraid to step outside your box in the kitchen. Variety is the spice of life! Try to incorporate a few new Belly Buddies. You may just fall in love with some of these new-to-you foods.

Now that you have a good handle on how FODMAPs, carb-dense foods, and pro-inflammatory fats wreak havoc on your digestive health and weight management—and how carb-light, low-FODMAP, fiber- and magnesium-rich foods heal and trim your tummy—it's time to sink your teeth into the tastiest way to your flattest and happiest tummy ever.

Your Personal 21-Day Plan

Get clean and lean with this flexible 3-week diet

THREE WEEKS, THREE PHASES, A MULTITUDE OF BENEFITS

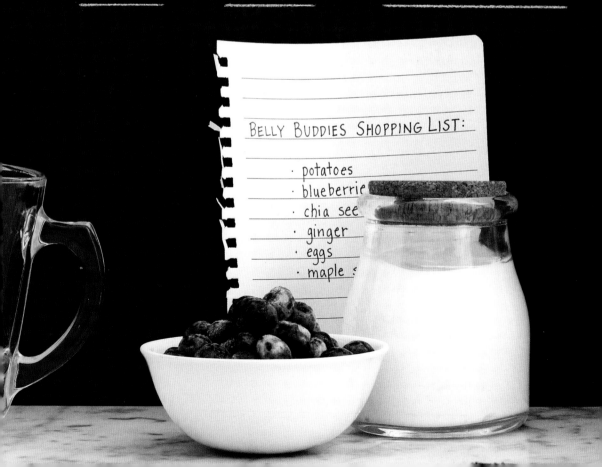

BELLY BUDDIES SHOPPING LIST:

- potatoes
- blueberrie[s]
- chia see[ds]
- ginger
- eggs
- maple s[yrup]

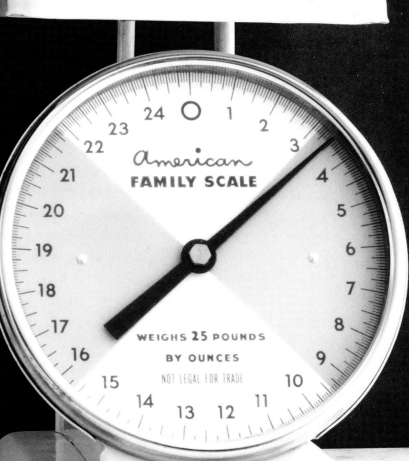

Chapter 3

Whether you are a newcomer or a 21-Day Tummy graduate, now is the time to create your *own* 21-day menu plan! Since we all have our own individual taste in food, this chapter will help you mix and match the recipes in this book with the right combination of foods to pacify your sensitive stomach while trimming your unwanted belly fat. These recipes and menus provide just the right balance of nutrients and tummy-taming ingredients to get at the root cause of your digestive discord and weight gain. It really boils down to two important things: balancing the bacteria that live in your intestines and reducing inflammation. Yes, finally a delicious nutrition plan that keeps you lean, maintains your energy, and stabilizes your GI symptoms for a lifetime!

The 21-Day Tummy plan incorporates the latest research on weight management and digestive health, and integrates this groundbreaking science into four simple rules. Eat:

1. **More magnesium-rich foods.** Magnesium deficiency is linked with inflammation and obesity. An estimated 68 percent of Americans are not getting enough of this essential mineral. Don't be one of them! Power up with magnesium-rich spinach, brown rice, pumpkin seeds, and peanut butter.

2. **More anti-inflammatory fats.** Healthy fats such as MUFAs specifically target visceral belly fat, and omega-3s combat inflammation. These anti-inflammation busters protect us from a slew of diseases, from heart disease to depression. And who doesn't love the idea of including olive oil, nuts, dark chocolate, and so many other deliciously healthful foods in their diet?

3. **Fewer carb-dense foods.** Foods with a high concentration of carbs per the weight of the food (think sugar, white flour, and most grains) are linked with inflammation. Replace them with

naturally carb-light foods, such as leafy greens, bananas, potatoes, lean meats, seeds, nuts, and olive oil, and a handful of what we call carb-light grains.

4. **Fewer FODMAPs.** FODMAPs are poorly absorbed sugars and fibers that feed our gut bacteria, causing excess gas. Many otherwise healthy foods contain FODMAPs, including apples, pears, watermelon, garlic, onions, and wheat. You'll minimize FODMAPs for the 21 days of the plan, then challenge each to see which ones you might be able to reintroduce. You'll learn more about these challenges in Appendix A.

Meal Planning Made Easy

The 21-Day Tummy diet consists of three phases, each designed with a special purpose. In all three phases, you'll enjoy three meals and a hearty snack. Once you get the hang of it, planning healthy, satisfying meals will become second nature. And the payoff for doing so is, of course, priceless—the trim and trouble-free tummy you've always wanted.

In all three phases, use the following guidelines to creating a balanced belly-friendly plate as a starting point.

- **Colorful veggies:** Fill half your plate with the Belly Buddy vegetables listed on page 26: green beans, carrots, kale, spinach, endive, arugula, Swiss chard, eggplant, parsnip, zucchini, and more. Pile on these nutrient-rich powerhouses! For the first 21 days of the plan, stick to those listed on page 26. After that, take the Belly Bully Tests described in Appendix A to learn which veggies your body is less sensitive to, so you can expand your personal repertoire of vegetables.

- **Fiber-rich carbs:** Fill one-quarter of your plate with fiber-rich, energy-boosting carbs. In Phase 1, stick with starchy vegetables like potatoes and sweet potatoes or fruits like bananas. In Phase 2, you can add low-FODMAP grains such as quinoa and oat bran to your options. In Phase 3, a larger selection of low-FODMAP grains are allowed, including corn tortillas, polenta, brown rice, and buckwheat. In general, keep these carb-rich food portions about the size of your fist.

- **Lean protein:** Fill the last one-quarter of your plate with eggs, tofu, tempeh, fish, seafood, and lean cuts of beef, pork, chicken, or turkey. Protein satisfies our tummy, so we feel full. Keep these portions to about the size of the palm of your hand or maybe a bit bigger for fish, which tends to be even lower in calories.

- **Healthy fats:** Accent your meal with healthy fats such as olive oil, walnuts, almonds, pine nuts, peanuts or peanut butter, chia seeds, flaxseeds, pumpkins seeds, avocados, and olives to fight inflammation. However, keep the portions small, such as 2 tablespoons walnuts, almonds, or peanut butter; 1 tablespoon olive oil; 5 to 10 olives; or ⅛ avocado. These portion sizes give you the health benefits but keep the calories and fat in check so you don't sabotage your weight loss efforts.

- **Sweet fruits:** Delight in the natural sweetness of wholesome fruits daily. Enjoy about 2 to 3 servings of whole fruit (1 serving might include 1 cup raspberries, strawberries, or blueberries, 1 small banana, or 1 orange). Hold the juice, which doesn't contain the all-important fiber!

In addition, follow these rules for best results:

- Avoid alcohol, which can irritate your digestive tract and contribute empty calories.

- Don't drink soda (it contains FODMAPs and carb-dense sugars), and avoid diet soda (it is full of artificial fake sugars); seltzer water is okay.

- Steer clear of caffeine if you have diarrhea; otherwise, a limited amount of caffeine is fine.

- Drink eight 8-ounce glasses of water per day.

- Stick to lactose-free milk.

- Space meals and snacks 2 to 3 hours apart.

In the guidelines that follow, you'll see that we suggest an approximate number of calories per day and per meal. These are designed to provide just enough calories and nutrition for a woman of average height and activity level to feel full and satisfied. Men, as well as taller and more active women, may find they need a little more. If that describes you, simply add more veggies to your day and/or add an extra snack. Whatever you do, don't starve yourself and don't go crazy trying to get your calorie counts (or carb densities or protein grams or anything else) to add up exactly. What's important is sticking to these general guidelines as much as possible and filling up on tummy-friendly Belly Buddies.

> Don't starve yourself and don't go crazy trying to get your calorie counts (or carb densities or protein grams or anything else) to add up exactly.

Please note that the quick-fix meals in the sample menus all make individual portions. However, the recipes in the book serve four (or sometimes more). We've done it this way so you can share the recipes with your family (if you usually cook for them), or you can freeze extra portions to use later. To be sure you are eating single servings, note the portion amount given with each recipe.

COMMON INGREDIENT SUBSTITUTIONS

If you are allergic to an ingredient called for in the meal plan, can't find it in the store, or simply hate it, here are some common substitutions you can make.

Lactose-free milk	Rice milk, light coconut milk†
Lactose-free cottage cheese	Farmer cheese (a low-lactose soft cheese), Greek yogurt (plain if using for dips)
Greens: kale, arugula, romaine, Swiss chard	Interchange as desired
Cabbage: green, red	Interchange as desired
Turnips	Parsnips, potatoes
Kiwi, star fruit	½ cup strawberries or blueberries
Papaya	Pineapple
Red quinoa	White or any other type of quinoa, brown rice
Chia seeds	Ground flaxseed or pumpkin seeds (pepitas)
Lean protein: fish, turkey breast or tenderloin, chicken breast, pork tenderloin, lean beef	Interchange as desired

†Rice milk and coconut milk are not preferred because they have less protein.

PHASE 1: FLATTEN (DAYS 1–5)

The lower calorie level in this phase (about 1,200 calories per day, or about 300 calories per meal or snack) will jump-start your weight loss while immediately soothing your sensitive digestive system. We ramp up your protein intake to ensure a full and satisfied tummy, including 80 to 90 grams over the course of the day. You'll enjoy a refreshing Belly Soother Smoothie (which was a favorite of many of our testers, including yours truly!) for one meal per day. (If you are especially sensitive to lactose, substitute a lactose-free yogurt for the Greek yogurt in the smoothies.) The focus of this phase is to nourish and calm your tummy with a selection of easy-to-digest foods. You'll go completely grain free (even the Belly Buddies oats, oat bran, quinoa, polenta, and buckwheat are not introduced until later) to quickly calm your GI symptoms. I found this phase the easiest to follow. You will feel lighter, leaner, and cleaner in just 5 days. You may also feel more energized and even keeled, as your body will be enjoying a balance of nutrient- and fiber-rich real foods that, of course, are gentle on the tummy.

How to Plan Phase 1 Menus

Since you'll have a Belly Soother Smoothie every day during this phase of the plan, I suggest you start by taking a look at the master recipe on page 85 and deciding what flavors and add-ins you want to try. If you find a version you really like, you can stick with that, but I encourage you to experiment with different fruit and vegetable combinations so you don't get bored. I like to start each day with a different variation.

Next, plan out your lunches and dinners. To cut down on shopping and prep time, you may want to select a couple of delicious soup and interesting salad recipes to make, and plan on eating some leftovers. If you choose one of our hearty Phase 1 soups in Chapter 5, which include protein, add some leafy greens on the side—perhaps with some sliced red peppers and baby carrots for more antioxidants, and topped with 2 teaspoons of one of our Basic Salad Dressings (page 54) as your source of healthy fats. If you select a Phase 1 salad from Chapter 7, have a piece of fresh fruit (such as a banana, orange, or kiwi), or try half a sweet potato on the side.

Alternatively, keeping the balanced belly-friendly plate in mind, you could pair a small portion of a protein-heavy Phase 1 main dish (Chapter 6) with a Phase 1 veggie side salad (Chapter 8) or side dish (Chapter 9). For your carbs, go with a baked white potato (about the size of your fist), with the skin on; half a baked sweet potato (about the same size); or a Belly Buddy fruit such as 1 cup of blueberries, a medium banana, or 1 cup of cantaloupe. At lunch, choose just one carb; at dinner, you can have both a potato and a fruit. (The slight reduction in carbs and calories at lunch will keep you satisfied, but will quell your digestive symptoms and allow for more rapid weight loss.) Or, you can keep it simple and pick one of the Phase 1 one-dish recipes in Chapter 7.

Finally, take a peek at the snack suggestions on page 77 and be sure to have the ingredients on hand for this all-important afternoon pick-me-up. It's imperative to pack a snack every day to ward off temptations to grab a cookie or head to the nearest vending machine.

Here are a few lunch and dinner combinations you can enjoy on this phase:

- *Provençal Fish Soup (page 120)* paired with a simple baby spinach salad topped with 10 baby carrots, 10 grape tomatoes, and 2 teaspoons of one of our Basic Salad Dressings (page 54)

- *Potato and Cheese Frittata (page 158)* enjoyed with 2 cups chopped summer squash sauteéd with 2 teaspoons sesame oil plus a small banana

- *Chicken Ambrosia (page 189)*

- *Margarita Shrimp Salad (page 202)* with an orange

Breakfast

Belly Soother Smoothie (page 85)

Lunch

Spinach, Pork, and Blueberry Salad (page 174) and a
handful of peanuts (about 20)

Snack

Dilly Cheese Dip: Mix ½ cup low-fat lactose-free cottage
cheese with a dash of dill (dry or fresh) and ground pepper.
Serve with 10 baby carrots and 5 cucumber slices.

Dinner

Balsamic Chicken: Grill, bake, or roast 3 ounces chicken
breast and drizzle with 1 teaspoon balsamic vinegar. Serve
with ½ sweet potato seasoned with a dash of cinnamon
and drizzled with 1 teaspoon olive oil. Have a green salad
(choose 2 cups spinach, arugula, or kale) topped with
2 teaspoons salad dressing (start with the *Basic Salad
Dressing (page 54)* and choose whichever variation you
like) and 1 tablespoon pepitas (hulled pumpkin seeds).
Enjoy with an orange.

Breakfast

Belly Soother Smoothie (page 85)

Lunch

Italian Chicken and Escarole Soup (page 112). Enjoy with
1 cup sliced strawberries and 10 almonds.

Snack

1 medium banana spread with 1 tablespoon peanut butter

Dinner

Roast Pork and Winter Vegetables (page 172). Serve with
2 cups steamed green beans dressed with 2 teaspoons
salad dressing (start with the *Basic Salad Dressing (page
54)* and choose whichever variation you like). Enjoy with
20 red grapes.

PHASE 2: SOOTHE AND SHRINK (DAYS 6–15)

For the next 10 days, you'll maximize belly fat loss by boosting anti-inflammatory foods rich in magnesium and monounsaturated fatty acids. You'll continue to enjoy one Belly Soother Smoothie per day, but your other meals will be larger and your calorie allotment a bit higher (about 1,400 calories per day, or about 350 calories per meal or snack) to keep your metabolism buzzing. Kate has bumped up your protein goal a bit, too; aim for about 100 grams a day to maintain your lean muscle and keep your digestion humming (remember that all your digestive enzymes are proteins).

In Phase 2, we introduce magnesium-rich quinoa and oat bran, the most carb-light of grains. You'll find that combining magnesium-rich fruits, veggies, nuts, and seeds, plus MUFA-rich oils, with these carb-light grains is a delicious way to lose belly fat.

> You'll find that combining magnesium-rich fruits, veggies, nuts, and seeds, plus MUFA-rich oils, with these carb-light grains is a delicious way to lose belly fat.

How to Plan Phase 2 Menus

You have a bit more wiggle room in the diet as you move from Phase 1 to Phase 2. Now that oat bran and quinoa have been added to your repertoire, try the *Quinoa and Oat Bran Cereal (page 93)* or perhaps the *Breakfast Fruit Salad (page 99)* for breakfast; enjoy your Belly Soother Smoothie at lunch instead. Alternatively, you can continue to have your smoothie for breakfast and plan a heartier lunch instead.

For lunch or dinner in this phase, remember that you can enjoy any of the Phase 2 as well as the Phase 1 recipes. Just keep the balanced belly-friendly plate in mind as you combine recipes to make sure you get twice as many veggies as you do carbs and protein. If you choose to forgo the recipes and create your own menu, start with half a plate of colorful Belly Buddy veggies topped with a drizzle of olive oil, a couple tablespoons of chopped nuts, a small handful of olives, or ⅛ avocado. Then add a lean protein source (about the size of your palm), such as a boneless, skinless chicken breast; flank steak or fish fillet (the fish can be a little bit bigger). Finally, enjoy a small baked white potato, half a sweet potato, or a fist-size portion of quinoa (about 1 cup). Be sure to include 2 to 3 fruit servings over the course of the day and one hearty snack per day.

Here are some lunch and dinner combos for you to try:

- *Italian Tomato and Meatball Soup (page 115)* with an orange and 10 almonds

- *Red Quinoa Burger with Tzatziki (page 161)* with baby spinach, red bell peppers, and baby carrot salad with 2 teaspoons dressing

- *Beef and Cabbage Stir-Fry with Sesame Quinoa (page 170)* and a kiwi

- *Asian Chicken Salad with Peanut Dressing (page 192)* and 1 medium roasted red potato drizzled with 1 teaspoon olive oil. Enjoy with 1 cup blueberries

Breakfast

Potato, Ham, and Cheddar Hash (page 89). Serve with
¾ cup fresh blueberries sprinkled with 2 tablespoons sliced
almonds.

Lunch

Belly Soother Smoothie (page 85)

Snack

Crunch and Go!: 10 almonds, 10 baby carrots, and a
reduced-fat mozzarella cheese stick

Dinner

Flavor-full Fish!: Grill or bake 6 ounces tilapia, haddock,
or cod seasoned with dill and juice of a lemon wedge.
Serve with a baked or grilled medium red-skinned potato
topped with 1 tablespoon each Greek yogurt and chopped
chives. Have an arugula salad: 2 cups arugula drizzled
with 2 teaspoons salad dressing (start with the *Basic Salad
Dressing (page 54)* and choose whichever variation you
like). Enjoy with a banana and 10 nuts (any kind except
pistachios or cashews).

Breakfast

Belly Soother Smoothie (page 85)

Lunch

Greek Quinoa and Chicken Salad: Roast, bake, or grill 4 ounces boneless, skinless chicken breast (or buy unseasoned cooked chicken, about ½ cup). Toss 1 cup cooked quinoa with 2 teaspoons salad dressing (start with the *Basic Salad Dressing (page 54)* and choose whichever variation you like), 10 grape tomatoes, 5 cucumber slices, 2 tablespoons feta cheese, and 2 tablespoons chopped nuts (any kind except pistachios or cashews). Top with the chicken (slice or shred first). Enjoy with 1 cup sliced strawberries.

Snack

Carrot Cake Parfait: Layer ½ cup nonfat vanilla Greek or lactose-free yogurt—or add 1 teaspoon vanilla extract or paste to ½ cup nonfat plain Greek or lactose-free yogurt—with ¼ cup grated carrots, 1 tablespoon chopped walnuts, and a sprinkle of cinnamon.

Dinner

Hazelnut-Stuffed Pork Chops (page 132). Serve with ½ medium sweet potato, baked and seasoned with 1 teaspoon olive oil and a dash of sea salt and pepper, and 1 medium zucchini, sliced and sautéed in 1 teaspoon sesame oil.

PHASE 3: BALANCE (DAYS 16–21)

This final phase emphasizes balance: balanced gut flora through a balanced plate. A combination of low FODMAP whole grains, lean protein, colorful veggies, and healthy fats are the ideal blend for weight management and stable blood sugar and insulin levels, not to mention out-of-the-ballpark energy levels and the calmest belly you have ever experienced.

Research indicates that the best mix to decrease inflammation and improve digestion includes about 40 percent carbs, 30 percent protein, and 30 percent fat.[1] Luckily, thanks to the balanced belly-friendly plates you've been enjoying, you already know how to achieve this optimal combination. Kate recommends that you stick with this basic mix for life. That being said, of course, we don't expect you to be calculating your protein, carb, and fat grams; just stay close to the proportions in the balanced plate, and you'll be fine. Kate has kept the calorie level at 1,400 per day (about 350 per meal or snack) to allow for continued weight loss. Protein-rich foods are encouraged at each meal to keep your belly content, with a goal of 100 grams of protein per day.

In Phase 3, we add in small portions of low-FODMAP grains, including oats, buckwheat, polenta, and brown rice. These boost the brain chemical serotonin, which stabilizes your mood without derailing your weight loss or destabilizing your tummy. You won't be having the Belly Soother Smoothie every day, but feel free to sub it in for a meal occasionally if you enjoy it!

How to Plan Phase 3 Menus

Continue to follow the balanced belly-friendly plate guidelines we introduced on page 59 to get the optimal mix of fiber-rich carbs, lean protein, fresh produce, and healthy fats.

For breakfast, this might mean a hearty hot cereal made with both oat bran and rolled oats (fiber-rich carbs), mixed with lactose-free milk (protein), and topped with fresh strawberries and blueberries (colorful produce) and 2 tablespoons of chopped nuts (healthy fats). Or try a hearty frittata cooked in olive oil (healthy fat) with a mix of shredded potatoes (fiber-rich carbs), eggs or egg whites (lean protein), and spinach and red pepper (colorful veggies), and served with an orange (fruit).

As a lunch or dinner option, enjoy a rice bowl: a scoop of warmed brown rice (fiber-rich carbs), topped with fresh spinach leaves, baby carrots, sliced cucumber, and cherry tomatoes (colorful veggies); grilled shrimp (lean protein); and a drizzle of balsamic vinegar and olive oil (healthy fat). If you're in the mood for pasta, try a fist-size portion of cooked brown rice pasta (fiber-rich carbs) topped with a drizzle of *Roasted Garlic Oil (page 54)* (healthy fats); a medley of colorful veggies such as spinach, zucchini, red peppers, and summer squash; and grilled chicken (lean protein). Serve 1 cup blueberries and strawberries on the side. The healthiest of plates are very colorful!

> In this phase, we've included some desserts to satisfy your sweet tooth.

In this phase, you'll see that we've included some desserts to satisfy your sweet tooth. We've made some tweaks to reduce the carb density of your favorite treats. But because the cakes, cookies, and other baked goods still tend to be a little more carb-dense than the other foods on the 21-Day Tummy plan, we suggest that you enjoy them only every other day. On days you do have dessert, keep the rest of your meals especially carb-light; stick with lean protein and fresh produce and avoid grain, as in Phase 1.

Here are some more delicious Phase 3 breakfast options you can try:

- *Blueberry Corn Muffin (page 102)* and ¾ cup egg whites (about 5-6 eggs or buy commercial egg whites, without onion, in the dairy section of the grocery store) scrambled with ½ cup spinach or arugula and 1 teaspoon olive oil

(continued on page 74)

Dorothy Nuzzo, Age 55

LOST 6½ POUNDS and 2¼ BELLY INCHES IN 21 DAYS!

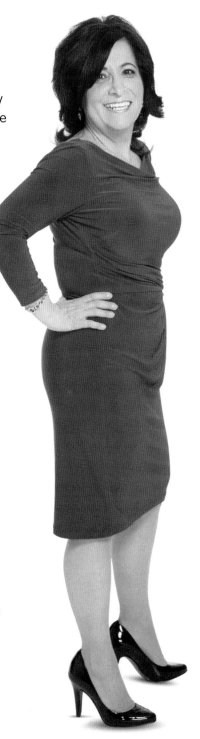

Like many women, Dorothy Nuzzo didn't like her belly very much. "It was big and in my way all the time," she complained before she started the 21-Day Tummy meal plan. When she sat, she felt the weight of her stomach pressing up, likely a cause of her frequent gas and heartburn. When she lay down to sleep, she found it tough to roll over. And every pound showed on her petite frame.

After 21 days? Heartburn and gas are no longer a part of Dorothy's life. They are 100 percent gone. Her body aches have decreased, she's more flexible, and she was able to go from 3.8 miles per hour on the treadmill to

Lightening— and Lighting—Up at Midlife

4.5 miles. "I feel much lighter," she says. "I can move much easier, [and] I feel much more comfortable in my clothes. I feel that my belly is a lot flatter." In addition, she exclaims, "I lost 6 pounds, and for someone my size—I'm only 4 foot 10 inches—that's a lot of weight. It shows right away." The best part? "I was always full. I never felt hungry, and I felt good about eating healthy foods."

(continued from page 72)

- *Savory Seeded Almond Breakfast Shortbread (page 101)* and ½ cup nonfat plain Greek or lactose-free yogurt mixed with 1 teaspoon vanilla extract and topped with 1 cup sliced strawberries

And here are a few Phase 3 lunch or dinner combos to get you started:

- *Tofu Coconut Curry (page 205)* and an orange

- *Pork, Kasha, and Kiwi Salad (page 178)* enjoyed with 2 cups steamed green beans sprinkled with 2 tablespoons sliced almonds

- *Deviled Chicken (page 145)* with a side salad: 2 cups kale or spinach greens, 10 baby carrots, 10 cherry tomatoes, and 2 teaspoons salad dressing; enjoy with 1 cup cantaloupe chunks

- *Turkey Braciole (page 149)* with 2 cups carrots sautéed in 1½ teaspoons olive oil and served with 1 cup fresh pineapple chunks

Breakfast

Green Eggs and Cheese: Microwave 4 large egg whites (about ½ cup) until light and fluffy (microwave for 30 seconds, then scramble with a fork, and cook for another 30 seconds, or until white and cooked through). Top with ½ cup baby arugula or spinach and ¼ cup finely shredded reduced-fat cheddar. The greens should wilt and the cheese should melt on the warm eggs; if not, put the plate back in the microwave for about 10 seconds. Enjoy with a banana spread with 1 tablespoon peanut butter.

Lunch

South of the Border Tortillas: Fill 2 warmed corn tortillas evenly with a mixture of ½ cup chopped (about 3 ounces) grilled, baked, or roasted chicken; 1 cup sliced bell peppers sautéed in 2 teaspoons olive oil and seasoned with a dash of (onion-free) chili powder and ¼ teaspoon cumin; and the juice of ½ lime. Enjoy with ¼ cup raspberries (about 15) and 10 almonds.

Snack

6 ounces nonfat plain Greek yogurt or lactose-free yogurt sweetened with 1 teaspoon maple syrup and topped with ½ cup blueberries, 1 tablespoon chopped nuts (any kind except pistachios and cashews), and 1 teaspoon chia seeds

Dinner

Barbecue-Glazed Flank Steak (page 129) and Strawberry **Balsamic Spinach Salad:** Top 2 cups baby spinach leaves with 1 cup sliced strawberries and 1 teaspoon chia seeds, and drizzle with 2 teaspoons olive oil, 1 teaspoon balsamic vinegar, and a dash of salt and pepper. Serve with ½ cup brown rice.

Breakfast:

Breakfast Fruit Salad (page 99) and a hard-cooked egg.

Lunch:

Savory Stuffed Potato: Bake 1 medium russet potato at 350 degrees for 50 minutes (or microwave for about 8 minutes, turning the potato over midway through cooking). Slice it in half lengthwise, drizzle with 2 teaspoons olive oil, and top evenly with ½ cup diced tomatoes, ½ cup chopped cooked chicken, and ¼ cup reduced-fat cheddar. Heat in the microwave for 30 seconds to 1 minute, or until the cheese is melted and the potato is warmed. Garnish with the green part of a scallion, drizzle with 1 teaspoon olive oil, and add a dash of salt and pepper. Enjoy with a kiwi.

Snack:

10 brown rice crackers, one mini cheese, and 10 chopped red pepper strips

Dinner:

Shrimp and Sautéed Zucchini Ribbons: Grill, boil, or roast 8 large shrimp. Scrub and rinse the skin of a medium zucchini. Using a vegetable peeler, create ribbons of the zucchini skin and flesh, discarding the seeded middle. Sauté the ribbons and 1 tablespoon pine nuts in a skillet with 2 teaspoons *Roasted Garlic Oil (page 54)* until both are slightly browned; remove from the heat and season with a drizzle of soy sauce. Serve with the shrimp and ½ cup cooked brown rice or quinoa.

Dessert:

One *Three-Citrus Coconut Macaroon (page 273)* and 1 cup nonfat lactose-free milk

TRIM AND TAME YOUR TUMMY ON THE GO

Life is busy! Cooking every meal, albeit wonderful in a perfect world, is not realistic with today's busy lifestyles. Plus many of us travel for business, making cooking as a nightly ritual impossible. To help you keep your tummy tame and waistline trim when dining away from home, here are a few suggestions:

Breakfast:
- Go for the plain oats. Add some fresh fruit and nuts.
- Choose an egg white omelet with veggies such as spinach or bell peppers and perhaps a small amount of cheese.
- Try a parfait with Greek yogurt or lactose-free yogurt, fruit, nuts, and a small amount of granola.
- If you are really dashing, grab a banana and a packet of peanut butter on the run.

Lunch or Dinner:
- Baked potato stuffed with sautéed veggies such as bell peppers, zucchini, summer squash, spinach, and a small amount of cheese
- Salmon, steamed spinach or green beans, and ½ sweet potato or medium white potato with a small amount of butter or a drizzle of olive oil
- Grilled chicken or shrimp cocktail, with a side salad dressed with balsamic vinegar and olive oil
- Petite filet mignon or flank steak, brown rice, and a garden salad

Just say no to:
- Fast foods
- All-you-can-eat buffets
- Fried foods

Satisfying Snacks

It's easy to derail your good eating track by simply allowing yourself to get over-hungry. I've been known to go for a chocolate from the office candy jar when I miss a meal or snack. While treats are okay occasionally, your best bet is to plan a healthful midday snack. Here are a few of my favorite snack inspirations. As with the recipes, remember that you can always have snacks from an earlier phase.

- **Carrot Cake Parfait:** Layer ½ cup nonfat vanilla Greek or lactose-free yogurt—or add 1 teaspoon vanilla extract or paste to ½ cup nonfat plain Greek or lactose-free yogurt—with ¼ cup grated carrots, 1 tablespoon chopped walnuts, and a sprinkle of cinnamon. (Phase 1)

- **Nutty Monkey:** Spread 1 tablespoon nut butter (peanut or almond) on a banana. (Phase 1)

- **Crunch and Go!:** Have 10 almonds, 10 baby carrots, and a reduced-fat mozzarella cheese stick. (Phase 1)

- **Dilly Cheese Dip:** Mix ½ cup low-fat lactose-free cottage cheese with a dash of dill (dry or fresh) and ground pepper. Serve with 10 baby carrots and 5 cucumber slices. (Phase 1)

- **Caprese Salad Bites:** Mix 1 mozzarella stick sliced into bite-size pieces with 10 cherry tomatoes, 1 tablespoon fresh basil slices, and a drizzle of balsamic vinegar. (Phase 1)

- **Tropical Surprise:** Mix together ½ cup diced pineapple (drained of juice) with 1 tablespoon sliced almonds, ¼ cup nonfat plain Greek yogurt or lactose-free yogurt, 1 tablespoon unsweetened shredded coconut, and a sprinkle of chia seeds. (Phase 1)

- **Roasted Chickpeas:** Drain and rinse canned chickpeas. Dry them on paper towels, add to a bowl, drizzle with 1 teaspoon olive oil and 1 teaspoon Dijon mustard, and stir to blend. Season with a dash of sea salt, pepper, and paprika. Place on a baking sheet in an even layer and roast at 400 degrees for 30 to 40 minutes, turning occasionally, until browned and crisp. Measure out ¼ cup chickpeas and enjoy with 10 baby carrots. (Phase 1)

(continued on page 80)

Gregg Roth, Age 47

**LOST 11½ POUNDS and
4½ BELLY INCHES IN
21 DAYS!**

Gregg Roth is feeling much more athletic. After the 21-Day Tummy plan, he reports, "I am able to play basketball a lot easier. I feel lighter on my feet and have less pain in my joints. I have more energy, and I feel less sluggish. I'm sleeping much better, too." It's amazing what a difference dropping 11½ pounds can make!

Plus, he says, "This diet was much better for digestion than other diets I've done. My digestion definitely im-

More Athletic and Happier in 3 Weeks!

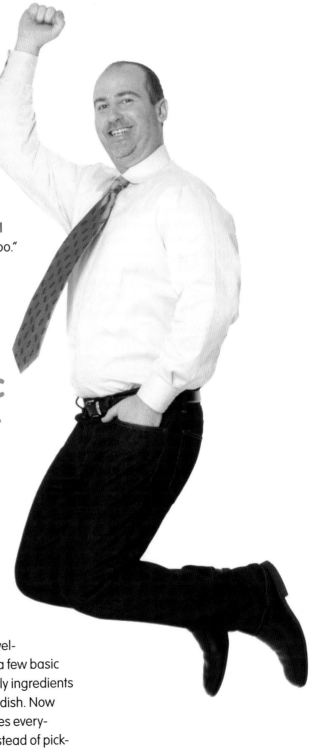

proved. I was in Florida for 5 days and went off the plan, and I could tell there was a huge difference in my digestive system. Let's just say it was a gas thing. That went away as soon as I went back on the plan."

After that experience, Gregg learned how to stick with the plan even while traveling. He learned he could always rely on a few basic meals and how to substitute belly-friendly ingredients when a restaurant didn't have a specific dish. Now he's in the habit of making healthy choices everywhere. "When I'm out at a restaurant, instead of picking the cheeseburger with fries, I'm getting vegetable main dishes and lean proteins and things like that."

(continued from page 78)

- **Peanut Butter Freeze:** Slice 1 small banana into 1½-inch slices. Mix ¼ cup nonfat plain Greek yogurt or lactose-free yogurt with 2 teaspoons almond or peanut butter. Dip the banana slices in the yogurt-peanut mixture and place on a plate lined with waxed paper. Freeze overnight, then enjoy this refreshing sweet treat! (Phase 1)

- **Blueberry Quinoa Yogurt Parfait:** Mix ½ cup nonfat plain Greek yogurt or lactose-free yogurt with 1 teaspoon maple syrup, ½ teaspoon vanilla extract, and a dash of cinnamon. Layer ¼ cup yogurt mixture with 2 tablespoons cooked quinoa and ¼ cup blueberries. Repeat layering one more time. (Phase 2)

- **Cheese Plate:** Enjoy 6 brown rice crackers, a reduced-fat or part-skim cheese stick, and 10 grapes. (Phase 3)

- **Tortilla "Pizza" Bites:** Top 10 baked tortilla chips evenly with ½ cup plain diced tomatoes (drained of juices), ¼ cup finely shredded part-skim mozzarella cheese, and sprinkle of oregano; melt in the microwave for about 15 seconds. (Phase 3)

- **Soothing and Satisfying "Hummus" Dip:** Blend 1 can chickpeas, drained and rinsed, with 1 tablespoon lemon juice, 1 teaspoon cumin, 1 tablespoon *Roasted Garlic Oil (page 54)*, and 1–2 tablespoons water to desired dip consistency. Enjoy ¼ cup of the dip with 10 baked corn tortilla chips and 10 baby carrots. (Phase 3)

✳✳✳

Menu planning only works if you work it around your schedule. Select more time-consuming recipes to make when your calendar is a little less busy, and go for the quick-and-easy recipes when you know you are on a time crunch. It's so much easier to plan a meal when you have the ingredients on hand. So review what recipes you will try this week, and what you will pair them with, and create a detailed grocery list to ensure you have what you need at your fingertips. Some recipes can be prepared on the weekend and frozen as a quick grab-and-go option during the workweek, too. When it comes down to any successful task in life, it really is all about the planning.

Learning how to balance your menus to include key nutrients to ease whole body inflammation and add equilibrium to your inner microbial ecosystem will lead to a leaner and happy life. The goal of healthy eating is to feel your best. I know you will enjoy and feel terrific eating the nourishing and tasty foods we have created for you and your sensitive tummy!

Now is the time to explore the amazing recipes we have included in the cookbook. We asked the best recipe developers in the business, Kate Slate and Sandy Gluck, to help create some delicious concoctions for you. Have fun cooking and eating these wonderful meals!

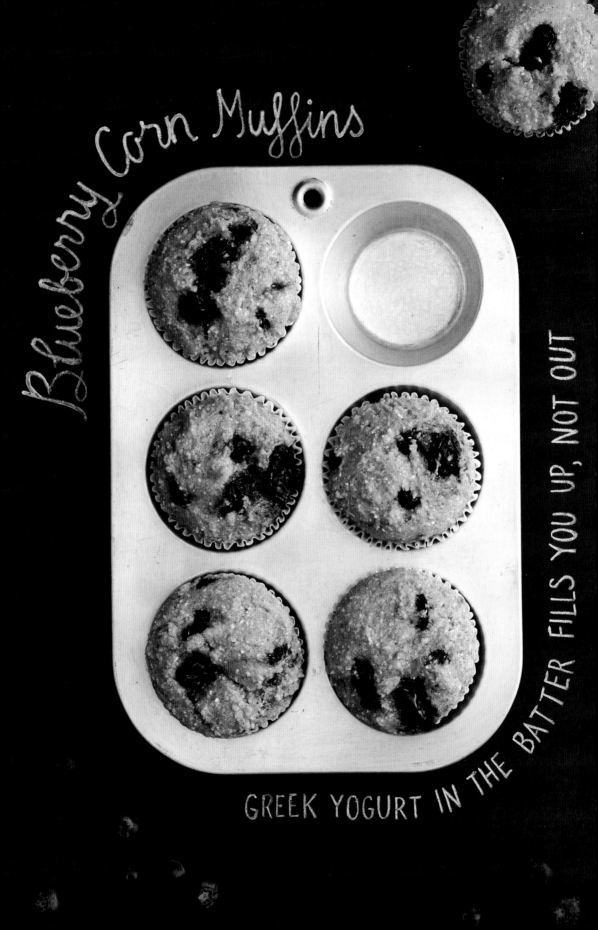

Blueberry Corn Muffins

GREEK YOGURT IN THE BATTER FILLS YOU UP, NOT OUT

Chapter 4

Breakfasts

BEAT
BLOAT
ALL
DAY
LONG

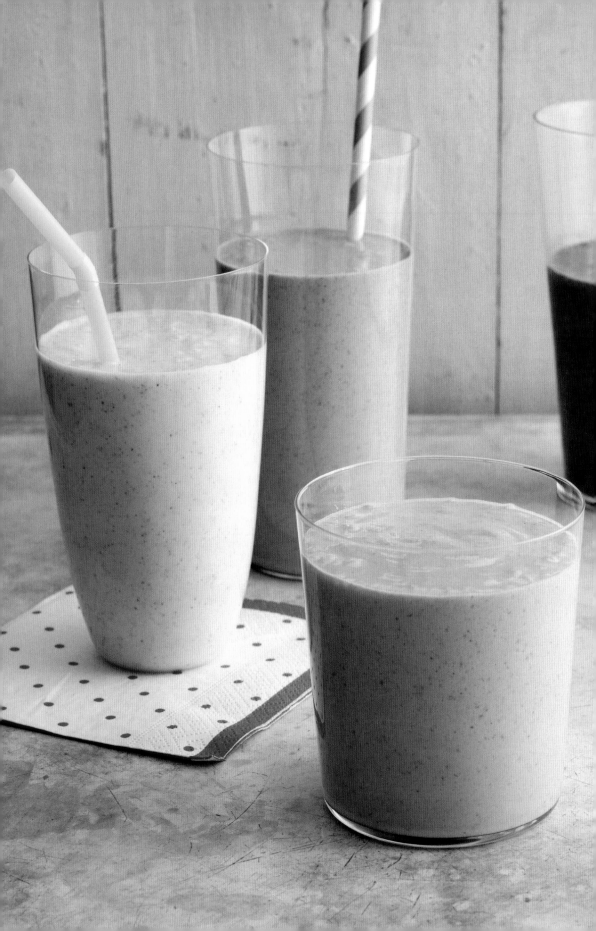

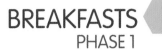
Belly Soother Smoothie

Hands-On Time: 5 minutes | **Total Time:** 5 minutes | **Makes:** 1 smoothie

A key component of the 21-Day Tummy diet, this satisfying smoothie includes creamy, protein-rich Greek yogurt and coconut milk plus different combinations of fruits (or vegetables), magnesium and fiber boosters, and MUFAs that keep your tummy and your taste buds happy!

Master Recipe

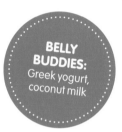

BELLY BUDDIES: Greek yogurt, coconut milk

- 6 ounces nonfat plain Greek yogurt
- 2 tablespoons light coconut milk
- 1–2 tablespoons water (frozen fruit requires more water than fresh)
- 1 teaspoon pure maple syrup (optional, for an extra hint of sweet)
- 4–6 ice cubes, or more, to create desired thickness (if using frozen fruits, omit ice)

Add one of each from the following groups.

Fruit or Vegetable

- 1 banana
- 1 cup strawberries
- 1 orange
- 2 kiwis
- ¾ cup blueberries
- ¾ cup raspberries
- 20 red grapes
- ½ cup cubed papaya
- ½ cup pineapple chunks
- ½ cup chopped kale leaves
- ½ cup chopped spinach
- ½ cup diced cucumber

Magnesium and fiber booster:

- 1 tablespoon chia, flax, or pumpkin seeds

MUFAs

- 1 teaspoon peanut butter
- 1 teaspoon almond butter

Flavoring (choose one or more, if desired):

- 1 teaspoon unsweetened cocoa
- ½ teaspoon vanilla extract
- ¼ teaspoon ground cinnamon
- ⅓ teaspoon ground ginger, or 1 teaspoon grated or minced fresh ginger
- 1 tablespoon fresh lemon juice (about ½ lemon)

Per serving (a typical shake): 281 calories • 20g protein • 8.5g fat (2g saturated) • 9g fiber • 35g carbohydrate • 79mg sodium • 59mg magnesium

If you are lactose intolerant: Reduce the yogurt to 4 ounces and up the coconut milk to 4 tablespoons. Or substitute lactose-free yogurt.

If you have gluten issues: Choose gluten-free brands of Greek yogurt and chia seeds.

Combine all of the ingredients in a blender and blend until frothy. Enjoy immediately.

(continued on page 86)

Belly Soother Smoothie *(continued from page 85)*

Here are a few new smoothie flavor combinations to get you started!

Raspberry Vanilla Creamy and refreshing

- 6 ounces nonfat plain Greek yogurt
- 2 tablespoons light coconut milk
- 1 teaspoon pure maple syrup
- ¾ cup raspberries
- 1 tablespoon chia seeds
- 1 teaspoon peanut butter
- 1 teaspoon vanilla paste or extract (paste infuses more vanilla flavor)

Tropical Crush Flavors of paradise await you!

- 6 ounces nonfat plain Greek yogurt
- 2 tablespoons light coconut milk
- 1 teaspoon pure maple syrup
- ¼ cup frozen pineapple chunks
- ½ banana
- 1 tablespoon chia seeds
- 1 teaspoon almond butter
- 1 teaspoon vanilla paste or extract
- 1–2 tablespoons water
- 4–6 ice cubes

Cinnamon Chocolate Velvety with hints of chocolate, cinnamon, and almonds

- 6 ounce nonfat plain Greek yogurt
- 2 tablespoons light coconut milk
- 1 teaspoon pure maple syrup
- 1 frozen banana
- 1 teaspoon unsweetened cocoa
- ¼ teaspoon ground cinnamon
- 1 teaspoon almond butter
- 1 tablespoon chia seeds (could sub flax)
- 2 tablespoons water
- 4–6 ice cubes

Blueberry Kale A burst of blueberry goodness

- 6 ounces nonfat plain Greek yogurt
- 2 tablespoons light coconut milk
- 1 teaspoon pure maple syrup
- ¾ cup frozen blueberries
- ½ cup chopped kale leaves
- 1 tablespoon pumpkin seeds
- 1 teaspoon almond butter
- 1 tablespoon fresh lemon juice (about ½ lemon)
- 1 tablespoon water
- 4–6 ice cubes

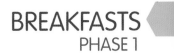
Tomato and Mozzarella Egg "Pizza"

Hands-On Time: 15 minutes | **Total Time:** 30 minutes | **Makes:** 4 wedges

Pizza without the carb-dense crust! The protein-rich eggs and cheese provide 17 grams of satiating protein per serving in this Italian-inspired dish.

4 large eggs

2 large egg whites

2 teaspoons water

½ teaspoon salt

2 teaspoons olive oil

1 cup shredded part-skim mozzarella cheese (4 ounces)

2 tablespoons grated Parmesan cheese

½ pound plum tomatoes, diced (1 cup)

¼ cup chopped fresh basil

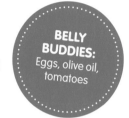

BELLY BUDDIES: Eggs, olive oil, tomatoes

1. Preheat the oven to 375°F.

2. In a large bowl, whisk together the whole eggs, egg whites, water, and salt. In a large nonstick ovenproof skillet, heat the oil over medium heat. Add the egg mixture and cook for 3 minutes, or until set around the edges.

3. Top with the mozzarella, Parmesan, tomatoes, and basil. Place in the oven and bake for 10 to 12 minutes, or until the eggs are set and the cheese has melted.

4. Run a metal spatula around the edge of the pan and slide the "pizza" onto a serving plate before cutting into wedges. Or serve the wedges right out of the pan.

Per wedge: 194 calories • 17g protein • 12g fat (5g saturated) • 0.5g fiber • 4g carbohydrate • 600mg sodium • 23mg magnesium

Cooking for One: Make the whole "pizza" and save for several lunches. Or make a smaller pizza: Use 2 large eggs, 1 egg white, 1 teaspoon water, ¼ teaspoon salt, ½ cup mozzarella, 1 tablespoon Parmesan, 1 large plum tomato, and 2 tablespoons basil. Heat 1 teaspoon oil in a small skillet and cook as described. Have half for breakfast and the remainder either for another breakfast or for lunch.

Breakfast Tortilla Cups

Hands-On Time: 20 minutes | **Total Time:** 25 minutes | **Makes:** 4 servings

You can make the tortilla cups well in advance. Store them airtight at room temperature for a week. Opting for reduced-fat cheeses decreases harmful saturated fat and calorie intake.

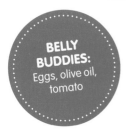

BELLY BUDDIES: Eggs, olive oil, tomato

Olive oil cooking spray

4 (6-inch) corn tortillas

¼ cup plus 2 tablespoons shredded reduced-fat Mexican blend cheese

4 large eggs

4 large egg whites

⅓ cup coarsely chopped fresh cilantro

½ teaspoon salt

¼ teaspoon black pepper

2 teaspoons extra-virgin olive oil

1 plum tomato, coarsely chopped

1. Preheat the oven to 375°F. Coat 4 cups of a jumbo muffin tin with cooking spray.

2. Heat a medium skillet over medium heat until a drop of water sizzles. Add a tortilla and cook to heat and soften, 30 to 45 seconds, flipping once or twice. While still hot and flexible, place it over one of the muffin cups and gently push it down into the cup. Repeat with the remaining 3 tortillas.

3. Spray the tortillas with cooking spray. Place in the oven and bake for 10 to 12 minutes, or until golden and crisp. Sprinkle the cheese evenly in the bottom of the tortilla cups.

4. Meanwhile, in a medium bowl, whisk together the whole eggs, egg whites, cilantro, salt, and pepper. In a large nonstick skillet, heat the oil over medium heat. Add the egg mixture and scramble to your preferred doneness.

5. Transfer the tortilla cups to plates and divide the hot eggs among them. Serve topped with the chopped tomatoes.

Per serving: 206 calories • 15g protein • 11g fat (3g saturated) • 1.5g fiber • 14g carbohydrate • 350mg sodium • 29mg magnesium

Cooking for One: Bake a single tortilla cup. In a small bowl, whisk together 1 large egg, 1 large egg white, 1 tablespoon chopped cilantro, ⅛ teaspoon salt, and a pinch of black pepper. Cook in ½ teaspoon oil in a small nonstick skillet. Fill a baked tortilla cup with 1½ tablespoons of the cheese and top with the eggs. Garnish with 4 grape tomatoes, chopped.

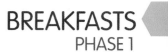

Potato, Ham, and Cheddar Hash

Hands-On Time: 10 minutes | **Total Time:** 30 minutes | **Makes:** 4 (1-cup) servings

Uncured ham has no nitrites and is generally lower in sodium than regular ham as well as some "low-sodium" hams. Compare brands when you're at the deli counter.

- 1¼ pounds large Yukon Gold potatoes
- 1 tablespoon plus 1 teaspoon extra-virgin olive oil
- ¼ pound uncured Black Forest ham, finely diced
- 1 cup frozen green peas, thawed

- ¼ teaspoon salt
- ¼ teaspoon black pepper
- Pinch of ground allspice
- ½ cup shredded reduced-fat cheddar cheese

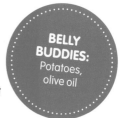

BELLY BUDDIES: Potatoes, olive oil

1. Poke a couple of holes in the potatoes and place in a microwave. Cook for 6 to 8 minutes, or until just barely fork-tender. When cool enough to handle, cut them into ⅓-inch cubes.

2. In a large nonstick skillet, heat the oil over medium-high heat. Add the potatoes and ham and toss to combine. Add the peas and sprinkle with the salt, pepper, and allspice. Toss again, then press the hash into an even layer.

3. Reduce the heat to medium, cover, and cook, without stirring, for 10 minutes, or until the potatoes on the bottom are lightly browned.

4. Remove from the heat, sprinkle with the cheese, re-cover, and let sit for 1 minute to melt the cheese. Serve straight out of the pan.

Per serving: 246 calories • 14g protein • 8.5g fat (3g saturated) • 4.5g fiber • 29g carbohydrate • 628mg sodium • 40mg magnesium

If you have gluten issues: Choose a gluten-free brand of ham.

Cooking for One: Make the whole batch and save for future breakfasts (or even lunch). It will keep quite well in the refrigerator for at least 5 days.

Poached Eggs and Grits

Hands-On Time: 20 minutes | **Total Time:** 20 minutes | **Makes:** 4 servings

The combo of creamy cheese grits topped with a soft egg makes for the perfect breakfast. Poaching eggs is an easy way of cooking them, if you just follow a couple of simple rules: Have the water simmering, not boiling, with a little bit of vinegar, and slide the eggs into the water one at a time. Spinach is rich in magnesium, iron, beta-carotene, potassium, and fiber!

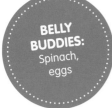

BELLY BUDDIES:
Spinach, eggs

2⅔ cups water

½ teaspoon salt

⅔ cup grits

⅔ cup shredded reduced-fat cheddar cheese

2 cups packed baby spinach (2 ounces), shredded

1 tablespoon distilled white vinegar

4 large eggs

1. In a medium saucepan, bring the water and the salt to a boil over medium heat. Add the grits and cook, stirring frequently, for 10 minutes, or until tender.

2. Stir in the cheese and spinach and remove from the heat.

3. Bring a large skillet of water to a simmer over medium-low heat. Add the vinegar. Crack each egg into a cup and then, at the edge of the pan, tip the egg into the simmering water. Cook, spooning some of the hot water over the eggs, for 3 minutes, or until the whites are set.

4. With a slotted spoon, scoop the eggs out one at a time and blot them on paper towels or a kitchen towel to get rid of excess water.

5. Divide the grits among 4 plates and top each with a poached egg.

Per serving: 223 calories • 12g protein • 8g fat (3.5g saturated) • 1.5g fiber • 25g carbohydrate • 506mg sodium • 6mg magnesium

Cooking for One: In a small saucepan, heat ⅔ cup water with ⅛ teaspoon salt and add 2 tablespoons plus 2 teaspoons grits and cook as directed. Stir in 2 tablespoons plus 2 teaspoons cheese and ½ cup shredded spinach. Poach 1 egg in a small skillet of simmering water (with ¾ teaspoon vinegar added to it).

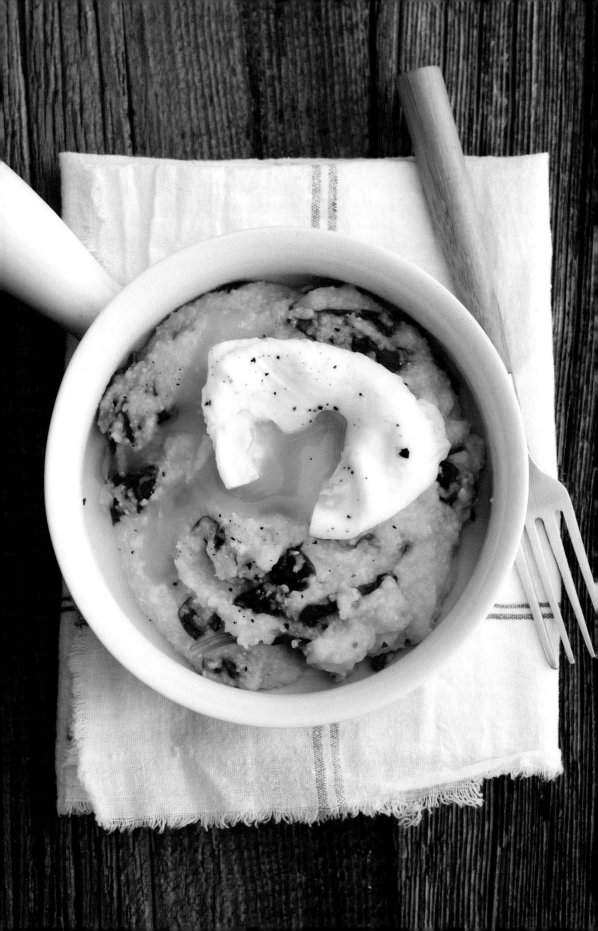

Breakfast Sliders

Hands-On Time: 10 minutes | **Total Time:** 15 minutes | **Makes:** 4 (2-slider) servings

You can certainly find roasted red peppers packed in jars in the supermarket or at the salad bar. But roasting your own is easy, and you can control the sodium levels: Cut the sides of the peppers into flat panels, place them skin side up under the broiler, and broil until charred (7 to 10 minutes). Flip them skin side down on the pan to cool, then peel.

BELLY BUDDIES:
Bell pepper, lean pork, ginger

½ cup roasted red pepper
¾ pound lean ground pork
½ teaspoon salt
½ teaspoon crumbled dried rosemary
½ teaspoon rubbed sage

¼ teaspoon ground ginger
⅛ teaspoon cayenne pepper
8 small Japanese brown rice crackers (look for brands with no onions or garlic)

1. In a food processor, puree the roasted pepper and transfer it to a medium bowl. Add the pork, salt, rosemary, sage, ginger, and cayenne and mix gently to combine. Shape into 8 patties.

2. Preheat the broiler with the rack 4 inches from the heat. Place the patties on a baking sheet and broil, flipping them over halfway through the cooking, for 4 minutes, or until just cooked through.

3. Serve the sliders on rice crackers.

Per serving: 199 calories • 16g protein • 13g fat (4.5g saturated) • 0g fiber • 4g carbohydrate • 371mg sodium • 15mg magnesium

If you have gluten issues: Choose a gluten-free brand of rice crackers.

Cooking for One: Make the whole batch and set aside 2 for cooking and eating immediately. Freeze the remaining 6 patties in 2-slider portions. Thaw before broiling.

Quinoa and Oat Bran Cereal

Hands-On Time: 20 minutes | **Total Time:** 20 minutes plus soaking time | **Makes:** 6 (½-cup) servings

Rinsing the quinoa gets rid of the slightly bitter-tasting saponins (naturally occurring compounds that coat the grains) that can impede digestion. For convenience, choose a brand that is pre-rinsed, such as Bob's Red Mill or Ancient Harvest. For this recipe, we also soaked the quinoa, which shortens the cooking time and reduces the saponins at the same time. This cereal is a delicious way to boost magnesium in your diet! Quinoa, oat bran, and pumpkin seeds are three of our favorite magnesium-rich foods.

¾ cup quinoa

½ cup oat bran

2 cups unsweetened rice milk

¾ cup water

½ teaspoon salt

1 medium banana (6 ounces), cut into 16 slices

2 tablespoons pure maple syrup

1 tablespoon hulled pumpkin seeds (pepitas)

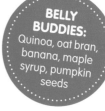

BELLY BUDDIES: Quinoa, oat bran, banana, maple syrup, pumpkin seeds

1. In a medium bowl, soak the quinoa in cold water for 30 minutes. Drain well and transfer to a medium saucepan.

2. Add the oat bran, rice milk, water, and salt to the pan and bring to a boil over medium heat. Reduce to a simmer, cover, and cook, stirring occasionally, for 15 minutes, or until the quinoa is tender.

3. Divide the hot cereal among 4 bowls and top each with 4 banana slices, 1½ teaspoons maple syrup, and ¾ teaspoon pumpkin seeds.

Per serving: 188 calories • 5g protein • 3g fat (0.5g saturated) • 3.5g fiber • 38g carbohydrate • 226mg sodium • 77mg magnesium

If you have gluten issues: Choose a gluten-free brand of oat bran.

Toasted Almond Oatmeal

Hands-On Time: 5 minutes | **Total Time:** 20 minutes | **Makes:** 4 (½-cup) servings

If you like this cereal, make a double or triple batch of the dry ingredients to have on hand. Oatmeal is a nutrient-dense whole grain and is rich in soluble fiber, which helps lower artery-clogging cholesterol.

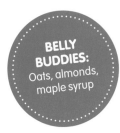

BELLY BUDDIES: Oats, almonds, maple syrup

½ cup quick-cooking oats

3 tablespoons slivered almonds

2¼ cups lactose-free 1% milk

½ cup water

¼ teaspoon vanilla extract

¼ teaspoon salt

Pinch of ground cinnamon (optional)

⅓ cup toasted brown rice couscous

4 teaspoons pure maple syrup

1. Preheat the oven to 375°F.

2. Spread the oats and almonds on a baking sheet and bake for 8 minutes, or until the almonds are lightly toasted.

3. Meanwhile, in a medium saucepan, combine 1¾ cups of the milk, the water, vanilla, salt, and cinnamon (if using). Bring to a simmer over medium heat. Stir in the couscous, partially cover, and cook at a low simmer (so the milk doesn't boil over) for 10 minutes.

4. Stir in the oats and almonds until well combined. Remove from the heat, cover, and let stand for 5 minutes.

5. Serve the cereal with the remaining ½ cup milk (2 tablespoons per serving) and a drizzle of maple syrup (1 teaspoon per serving).

Per serving: 197 calories • 8g protein • 5g fat (1g saturated) • 3g fiber • 31g carbohydrate • 216mg sodium • 34mg magnesium

If you have gluten issues: Choose a gluten-free brand of oats.

Cooking for One: Make the whole amount and refrigerate what you don't eat. For future breakfasts, scoop out ½ cup of the cereal and reheat with 2 or 3 tablespoons lactose-free milk in the microwave for about 45 seconds. Drizzle with 1 teaspoon maple syrup.

Crunchy Granola Bars

Hands-On Time: 10 minutes | **Total Time:** 20 minutes plus chilling time | **Makes:** 8 bars

Most commercial granola bars are made with added inulin (chicory root extract), which can contribute to belly bloating, but not these all-natural grab-and-go bars! However, check the label on "natural" peanut butters—they often have sugar added to them. These bars will keep for several days in the refrigerator, or can be wrapped individually and frozen for up to 3 months.

1 cup rolled oats

2 tablespoons hulled pumpkin seeds (pepitas)

1 tablespoon hulled sunflower seeds

¼ teaspoon salt

¼ cup natural creamy peanut butter

2 tablespoons pure maple syrup

2 tablespoons lactose-free 1% milk

Olive oil cooking spray

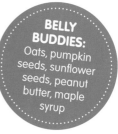

BELLY BUDDIES: Oats, pumpkin seeds, sunflower seeds, peanut butter, maple syrup

1. Preheat the oven to 425°F.

2 Place the oats on a small baking sheet and toast, stirring once, for 10 minutes, or until the oats are lightly browned. Transfer to a bowl and add the pumpkin seeds, sunflower seeds, and salt.

3. In a small saucepan, heat the peanut butter, maple syrup, and milk over low heat until the peanut butter has melted. Add it to the bowl with the oats mixture and toss until thoroughly coated.

4. Coat an 8 x 8-inch pan with cooking spray. Transfer the mixture to the pan and with dampened hands, press the mixture into the pan, smoothing the top. Refrigerate for 1 hour, or until firm, then cut into 8 bars.

Per bar: 123 calories • 4g protein • 6.5g fat (1g saturated) • 1.5g fiber • 12g carbohydrate • 75mg sodium • 17mg magnesium

If you have gluten issues: Choose a gluten-free brand of oats.

Toasted Oat Muesli with Peanuts and Grapes

Hands-On Time: 10 minutes | **Total Time:** 20 minutes plus soaking time | **Makes:** 6 (3/4-cup) servings

Muesli is an uncooked oat cereal developed in the 1900s by a Swiss physician as part of a diet designed to promote health. The oats (which we have toasted to give greater depth of flavor) are combined with peanuts, grapes, maple syrup, yogurt, and milk and then soaked to soften the oats. The result is both satisfying and filling.

BELLY BUDDIES: Oats, Greek yogurt, maple syrup, peanuts, grapes

1½ cups rolled oats
1½ cups lactose-free 1% milk
½ cup nonfat plain Greek yogurt
3 tablespoons pure maple syrup

¼ cup unsalted peanuts, chopped
12 seedless red grapes, quartered

1. Preheat the oven to 350°F. Place the oats on a baking sheet and toast for 10 minutes, or until fragrant, crisp, and lightly browned. Cool to room temperature.

2. In a medium bowl, whisk together the milk, yogurt, and maple syrup until combined. Add the toasted oats, peanuts, and grapes and stir until combined.

3. Refrigerate for at least 8 hours (or up to 12 hours) to soften the oats.

Per serving: 187 calories • 8g protein • 5g fat (1g saturated) • 3g fiber • 28g carbohydrate • 40mg sodium • 22mg magnesium

If you have gluten issues: Choose gluten-free brands of Greek yogurt and oats.

Cooking for One: Toast ¼ cup plus 2 tablespoons rolled oats and combine with 6 tablespoons lactose-free 1% milk, 2 tablespoons nonfat plain Greek yogurt, 2¼ teaspoons maple syrup, 1 tablespoon peanuts, and 3 grapes. Soak as directed.

Multigrain Pancakes

Hands-On Time: 20 minutes | **Total Time:** 20 minutes | **Makes:** 4 (2-pancake) servings

You can switch this recipe up by swapping in cornmeal for the almond flour and 2 large egg whites for the whole egg. If you like, you can mix together the dry ingredients and store them for up to several months at room temperature; when you're ready, add the other ingredients and you've got pancakes on the table in no time. Add a mashed banana or fold in a cup of blueberries to make these fiber-rich pancakes even healthier!

½ cup sorghum flour
¼ cup brown rice flour
2 tablespoons almond flour
2 tablespoons ground flaxseed
1½ teaspoons baking powder
¼ teaspoon salt

½ cup nonfat plain Greek yogurt
½ cup water
1 large egg
½ teaspoon vanilla extract
1 tablespoon extra-virgin olive oil

BELLY BUDDIES: Flaxseed, Greek yogurt, egg, olive oil

1. In a large bowl, stir together the sorghum flour, rice flour, almond flour, flax, baking powder, and salt.

2. In a separate bowl, whisk together the yogurt, water, egg, and vanilla. Stir into the flour mixture.

3. In a large nonstick skillet, heat the oil over medium heat. Drop the batter by 2 tablespoons to make 4 pancakes and cook for 2 minutes, or until bubbles appear on the surface. Carefully turn the pancakes over and cook for 2 minutes longer, or until the undersides are golden brown and the pancakes are cooked through.

4. Repeat with the remaining batter to make a total of 8 pancakes.

Per serving: 198 calories • 8g protein • 8g fat (1g saturated) • 3g fiber • 24g carbohydrate • 383mg sodium • 12mg magnesium

If you have gluten issues: Choose a gluten-free brand of baking powder and Greek yogurt.

Cooking for One: Cook the whole batch and freeze the pancakes in 2-pancake portions. To reheat, wrap in foil and bake at 350°F for 5 to 7 minutes, or until piping hot.

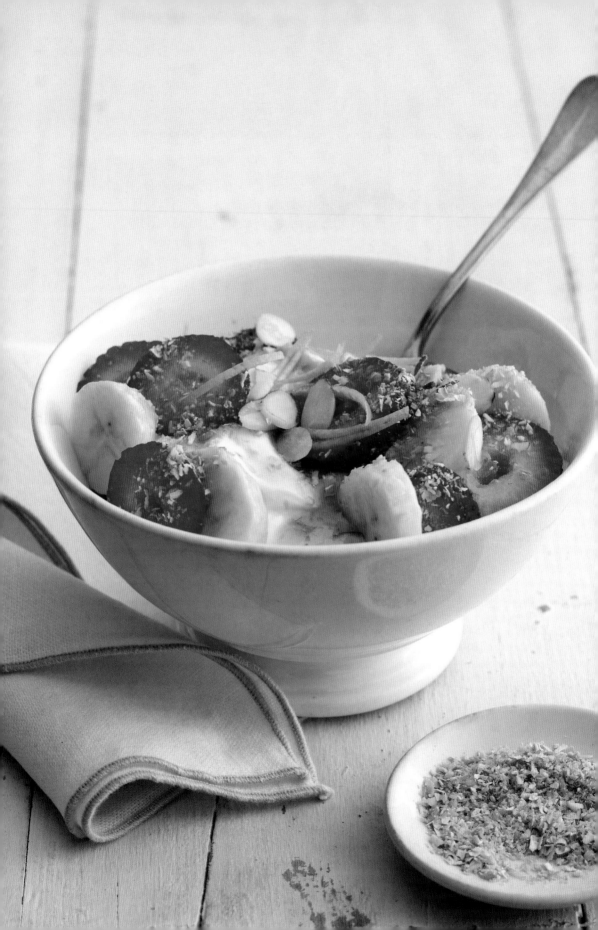

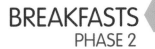

Breakfast Fruit Salad

Hands-On Time: 15 minutes | **Total Time:** 15 minutes | **Makes:** 4 (1-cup) servings

Every ingredient in this concoction is a Belly Buddy! Your digestive tract will love starting the day with this satisfying probiotic, antioxidant, magnesium-rich recipe. The yogurt mixture can be made up to 3 days ahead and refrigerated. If you'd like, swap in blueberries or raspberries for the strawberries.

1 cup nonfat plain Greek yogurt

½ teaspoon grated orange zest

¼ cup fresh orange juice

1 cup sliced strawberries

2 medium bananas, thickly sliced

1 tablespoon plus 1 teaspoon pure maple syrup

3 tablespoons oat bran

3 tablespoons ground flaxseed

2 tablespoons sliced almonds

BELLY BUDDIES: Greek yogurt, strawberries, bananas, maple syrup, oat bran, flaxseed, almonds

1. In a blender, combine the yogurt, orange zest, and orange juice. Puree until very smooth.

2. In a medium bowl, combine the strawberries and bananas, then divide among 4 bowls.

3. Drizzle 6 tablespoons yogurt dressing and 1 teaspoon maple syrup over each serving. Scatter the oat bran, flax, and almonds on top.

Per serving: 170 calories • 19g protein • 4g fat (0g saturated) •5g fiber • 30g carbohydrate • 23mg sodium • 43mg magnesium

If you have gluten issues: Choose gluten-free brands of Greek yogurt and oat bran.

Cheddar Scones

Hands-On Time: 15 minutes | **Total Time:** 45 minutes | **Makes:** 8 scones

Cayenne gives a slight kick to these hearty scones, but feel free to leave it out (or up it if you like things spicy). And you can swap in any reduced-fat cheese for the cheddar. Chia seeds and flaxseeds provide a source of plant-based omega-3 anti-inflammation–boosting healthy fats. The scones can be wrapped individually and frozen. To reheat, wrap in foil and heat in a 350°F oven for about 20 minutes.

BELLY BUDDIES: Oats, flaxseed, chia seeds, Greek yogurt, olive oil

1¾ cups rolled oats
⅓ cup ground flaxseed
1 tablespoon chia seeds
2 teaspoons baking powder
2 teaspoons light brown sugar
⅛ teaspoon cayenne pepper
½ teaspoon salt
⅔ cup nonfat plain Greek yogurt
2 tablespoons plus 1 teaspoon extra-virgin olive oil
¾ cup shredded reduced-fat cheddar cheese (3 ounces)

1. Preheat the oven to 425°F. Line a baking sheet with parchment paper.

2. Spread the oats on the baking sheet and bake, stirring once, for 10 minutes, or until toasted and lightly browned. Leave the oven on. Reserve the parchment-lined baking sheet.

3. Transfer 1½ cups of the oats to a food processor and pulse until finely ground.

4. In a large bowl, stir together the ground oats, flaxseed, chia seeds, baking powder, sugar, cayenne, salt, and the remaining ¼ cup toasted oats. With a pastry blender (or 2 knives used scissors fashion), cut in the yogurt and oil until the mixture resembles coarse crumbs. Stir in the cheese.

5. Transfer the dough to the parchment-lined pan and pat into a 9-inch round. Make 8 wedge cuts into the dough, cutting through but not separating the wedges (this will give you softer, more tender sides). Bake for 20 minutes, or until the top is golden brown and the scones are set. To serve, separate into wedges.

Per scone: 178 calories • 8g protein • 9.5g fat (2.5g saturated) • 3.5g fiber • 17g carbohydrate • 381mg sodium • 5mg magnesium

If you have gluten issues: Choose gluten-free brands of oats, chia seeds, baking powder, and Greek yogurt.

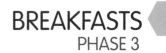

Savory Seeded Almond Breakfast Shortbread

Hands-On Time: 25 minutes | **Total Time:** 45 minutes plus cooling time |
Makes: 6 (2-wedge) servings

Have these with ½ cup nonfat plain Greek yogurt seasoned with 2 tablespoons chopped fresh dill, parsley, or basil. Or simply serve with a glass of lactose-free 1% milk.

Olive oil cooking spray
⅔ cup brown rice flour
¼ cup almond flour
½ cup grated Parmesan cheese
½ teaspoon salt
¼ teaspoon black pepper

2 tablespoons extra-virgin olive oil
1 tablespoon hulled sunflower seeds
2 teaspoons chia seeds
1 large egg white
2 tablespoons water

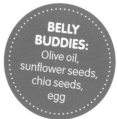

BELLY BUDDIES:
Olive oil, sunflower seeds, chia seeds, egg

1. Preheat the oven to 375°F. Coat a 9-inch springform pan or a tart pan with a removable bottom with cooking spray.

2. In a large bowl, combine the rice flour, almond flour, cheese, salt, and pepper. With a pastry blender (or 2 knives used scissors fashion), cut in the oil until the mixture forms coarse crumbs. Stir in the sunflower and chia seeds.

3. In a small bowl, whisk together the egg white and water and add to the flour mixture, stirring until blended. Transfer to the tart pan and with your hands, press the dough to the edges of the pan.

4. With a knife, deeply score into 12 wedges, cutting almost through to the bottom. Bake for 20 minutes, or until set. While still warm, cut through the shortbread where it was scored to separate the wedges and let cool in the pan.

Per serving: 180 calories • 6g protein • 11g fat (2g saturated) • 1.5g fiber • 16g carbohydrate • 309mg sodium • 25mg magnesium

If you have gluten issues: Choose a gluten-free brand of chia seeds.

Cooking for One: Make the whole batch and store leftovers in the freezer (they'll stay fresher than if you store them in the fridge). Wrap individually to freeze, then unwrap and thaw on the countertop.

Blueberry Corn Muffins

Hands-On Time: 10 minutes | **Total Time:** 30 minutes plus cooling time | **Makes:** 12 muffins

Adding Greek yogurt to muffin and bread recipes boosts protein and calcium content in the most delicious way. This is a great recipe to put together on the weekend so you have breakfast muffins all week long. Refrigerate the number of muffins you think you'll eat within 5 days and freeze the remainder. Reheat the frozen muffins in the microwave (1 to 2 minutes).

BELLY BUDDIES: Flaxseed, eggs, Greek yogurt, maple syrup, olive oil, blueberries

1 cup brown rice flour
1 cup yellow cornmeal
¼ cup ground flaxseed
2 teaspoons baking powder
1 teaspoon baking soda
½ teaspoon salt
¼ teaspoon ground cinnamon
2 large eggs
¾ cup nonfat plain Greek yogurt
½ cup pure maple syrup
3 tablespoons extra-light olive oil
1½ cups blueberries

1. Preheat the oven to 375°F. Line 12 cups of a muffin tin with paper liners.

2. In a mixer bowl, whisk together the rice flour, cornmeal, flax, baking powder, baking soda, salt, and cinnamon. Make a well in the center of the ingredients and add the eggs, yogurt, maple syrup, and oil. Mix on medium-low speed until just combined. Fold in the blueberries.

3. Divide the batter among the muffin cups. Bake, rotating the pan front to back halfway through, for 16 to 18 minutes, or until browned on top and a wooden pick inserted in the center of a muffin comes out clean. Transfer the muffins to a rack to cool.

Per muffin: 202 calories • 5g protein • 5.5g fat (1g saturated) • 2g fiber • 34g carbohydrate • 315mg sodium • 9mg magnesium

If you have gluten issues: Choose gluten-free brands of baking powder and Greek yogurt.

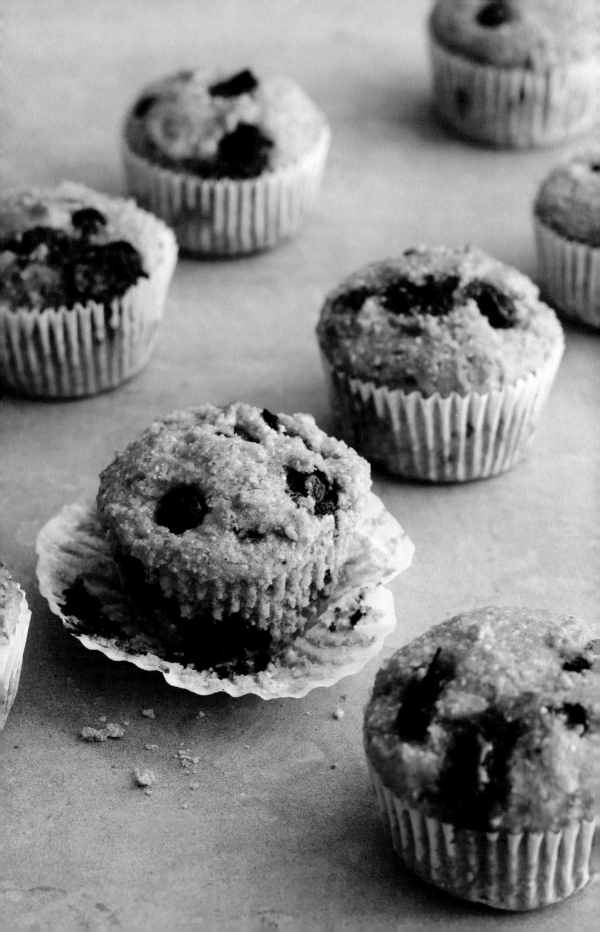

Italian Tomato & Meatball Soup

MADE WITH
BELLY-FRIENDLY
OATS AND CHIA SEEDS

Chapter 5

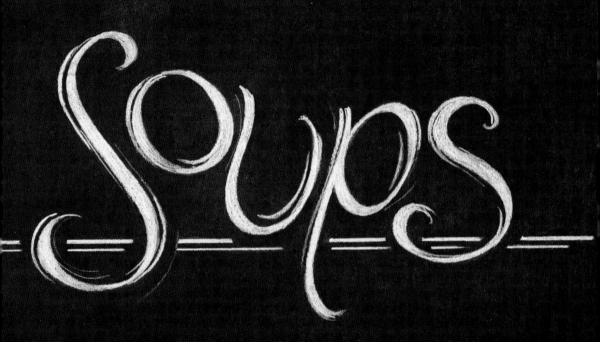

Soups

carb-light comfort food for your tummy

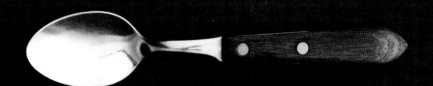

Beef Borscht

Hands-On Time: 30 minutes | **Total Time:** 45 minutes | **Makes:** 4 (1¾-cup) servings

Cabbage is a member of the cruciferous veggie family, well known for reducing cancer risk. Cabbage is also a staple of many weight-loss plans (remember the cabbage soup diet?) because it is super low-calorie—it has only 22 calories per cup! Plus, it provides 2 grams of fiber to keep you full and aid digestion. If you're planning on making this soup ahead, cook through step 2 and store in the fridge. Then when ready to serve, bring the soup back to a simmer and add the flank steak and vinegar.

BELLY BUDDIES: Olive oil, ginger, carrots, cabbage, tomatoes, lean beef

- 1 tablespoon extra-virgin olive oil
- 1 tablespoon minced fresh ginger
- 2 carrots, thinly sliced
- 1 beet (6 ounces), peeled, halved, and thinly sliced
- 2 cups shredded green cabbage
- 2 plum tomatoes, coarsely chopped
- 4 cups low-sodium beef broth (look for brands with no onions or garlic)
- ½ teaspoon salt
- ½ pound flank steak, thinly sliced across the grain, then cut into ½-inch-wide pieces
- 1 tablespoon red wine vinegar

1. In a large saucepan, heat the oil over medium heat. Add the ginger and cook, stirring, for 1 minute. Add the carrots, beets, cabbage, and tomatoes and cover. Cook, stirring occasionally, for 10 minutes, or until the carrots are crisp-tender.

2. Add the broth and salt and bring to a boil. Reduce to a simmer and cook for 15 minutes, or until the vegetables are very tender.

3. Add the flank steak and vinegar and simmer for 1 minute, or just until cooked through.

Per serving: 170 calories • 17g protein • 7g fat (1.5g saturated) • 3g fiber • 11g carbohydrate • 524mg sodium • 36mg magnesium

If you have gluten issues: Choose gluten-free brands of beef broth.

Cooking for One: Make the whole batch, and refrigerate or freeze the leftovers in 1¾-cup portions.

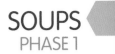

Smoky Lentil and Ham Soup

Hands-On Time: 10 minutes | **Total Time:** 45 minutes | **Makes:** 4 (1½-cup) servings

Lentils have fewer FODMAPs than most legumes, and canned lentils have the fewest. In addition, canned lentils are already cooked, making for a super quick soup. Seek out uncured ham at the deli. It has no nitrites or nitrates and is lower in sodium than cured ham.

4 cups low-sodium chicken broth (look for brands with no onions or garlic) or Homemade Chicken Broth (page 111)

1 can (14.5 ounces) no-salt-added fire-roasted diced tomatoes (look for brands with no onions or garlic)

2 teaspoons smoked paprika

½ teaspoon crumbled dried rosemary

1 can (15 ounces) lentils (look for brands with no onions or garlic)

1 large carrot, thinly sliced

2 ounces uncured ham, coarsely chopped

¼ teaspoon salt

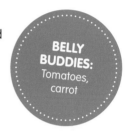

BELLY BUDDIES: Tomatoes, carrot

1. In a large saucepan, combine the broth, tomatoes, paprika, and rosemary and bring to a boil.

2. Stir in the lentils, carrot, ham, and salt. Reduce to a simmer, cover, and cook for 20 minutes, or until the carrots are tender.

Per serving: 155 calories • 13g protein • 0.5g fat (0g saturated) • 9.5g fiber • 23g carbohydrate • 458mg sodium • 4mg magnesium

If you have gluten issues: Choose gluten-free brands of chicken broth, ham, and paprika.

Cooking for One: Make the whole batch, and refrigerate or freeze the leftovers in 1½-cup portions.

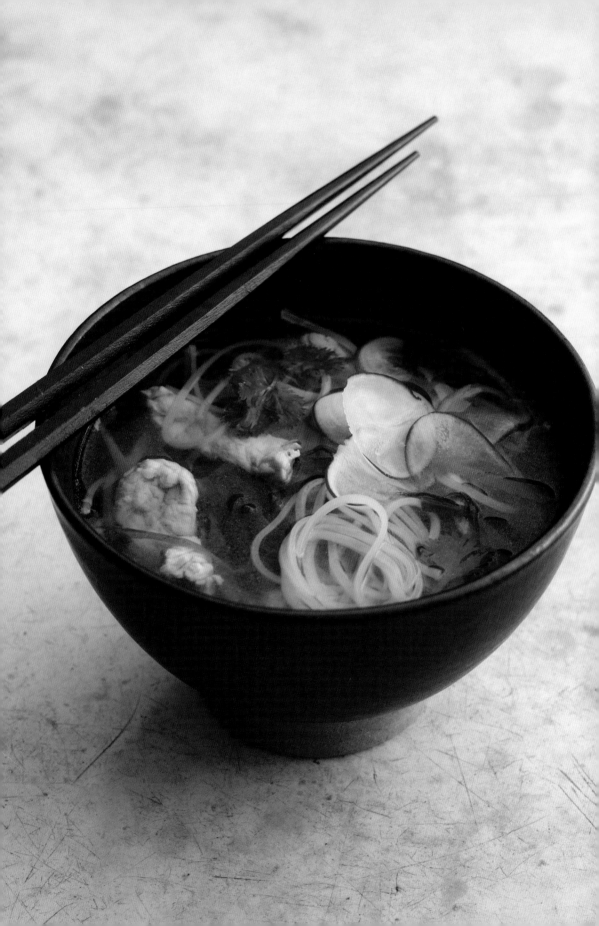

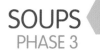

Pork and Ramen Soup

Hands-On Time: 15 minutes | **Total Time:** 25 minutes | **Makes:** 4 (2-cup) servings

Rice noodles can be found in the specialty section of most supermarkets. Once opened, store them as you would other types of pasta. The ginger in this recipe provides delicious flavor. It also has many medicinal qualities: It's known for quelling nausea and minimizing pain associated with arthritis and headaches.

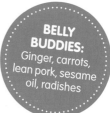

BELLY BUDDIES: Ginger, carrots, lean pork, sesame oil, radishes

- 4 cups low-sodium chicken broth (look for brands with no onions or garlic) or Homemade Chicken Broth (page 111)
- 2 cups water
- ½ cup sliced scallion greens or chives
- 3 tablespoons finely chopped fresh ginger
- 1 tablespoon reduced-sodium tamari or soy sauce
- ½ teaspoon salt
- 2 carrots, shredded
- 1½ ounces brown rice noodles
- ½ pound boneless pork loin chops, thinly sliced crosswise
- 2 tablespoons rice vinegar
- 1 tablespoon plus 1 teaspoon sesame oil
- 4 radishes, thinly sliced (½ cup)
- ¼ cup cilantro leaves

1. In a Dutch oven or 5-quart saucepan, bring the broth, water, scallion greens, ginger, tamari , and salt to a boil over high heat. Reduce to a simmer, cover, and cook for 5 minutes to concentrate the flavors.

2. Add the carrots and rice noodles and cook for 2 minutes, or until the noodles are tender. Add the pork and cook for 30 seconds, or until just cooked through. Remove from the heat and stir in the vinegar, sesame oil, radishes, and cilantro.

Per serving: 193 calories • 14g protein • 8.5g fat (2g saturated) • 2g fiber • 14g carbohydrate • 585mg sodium • 19mg magnesium

If you have gluten issues: Choose gluten-free brands of chicken broth and tamari.

Cooking for One: In a small saucepan, heat 1 cup broth with ½ cup water, 2 tablespoons scallion greens, 2 teaspoons ginger, ¾ teaspoon tamari, and ⅛ teaspoon salt. Add ½ carrot, ½ ounce rice noodles, 2 ounces pork, ½ teaspoon vinegar, 1 teaspoon sesame oil, 1 sliced radish, and 1 tablespoon cilantro leaves.

Chipotle Pork and Pepper Soup

Hands-On Time: 15 minutes | **Total Time:** 25 minutes | **Makes:** 4 (2-cup) servings

Chipotle peppers are smoked jalapeños, so the chipotle powder adds a subtle smoky flavor along with the heat. You could also make this soup with turkey breast in place of the pork loin. The tri-color peppers add vibrant color, flavor, a nice dose of immune-boosting vitamin C, and a variety of carotenoids, important disease-fighting plant pigments.

BELLY BUDDIES: Lean pork, olive oil, bell peppers, ginger

- ¼ cup potato starch
- ¾ pound center-cut boneless pork loin chops, cut into thin strips
- 4 teaspoons extra-virgin olive oil
- 1 yellow bell pepper, thinly sliced
- 1 red bell pepper, thinly sliced
- 1 orange bell pepper, thinly sliced
- 1 tablespoon slivered fresh ginger
- ½ plus ⅛ teaspoon salt
- 4½ cups low-sodium chicken broth (look for brands with no onions or garlic) or Homemade Chicken Broth (page 111)
- ½ teaspoon chipotle chile powder

1. Place the potato starch in a large bowl. Add the pork and toss to coat. Shake off and discard the excess potato starch.

2. In a large nonstick saucepan, heat 2 teaspoons of the oil over medium-high heat. Add the pork and cook for 2 minutes, or until mostly opaque but still pink in the center. Transfer the pork to a plate.

3. Add the remaining 2 teaspoons oil, the bell peppers, ginger, and ½ teaspoon salt to the saucepan and cook, stirring frequently, for 2 minutes, or until the peppers begin to soften.

4. Add the broth, chile powder, and remaining ⅛ teaspoon salt to the pan and bring to a boil. Reduce to a simmer, return the pork to the pan, and cook for 3 minutes, or just until the peppers are tender and the pork is cooked through.

Per serving: 303 calories • 29g protein • 13g fat (3.5g saturated) • 2g fiber • 15g carbohydrate • 573mg sodium • 41mg magnesium

If you have gluten issues: Choose a gluten-free brand of chicken broth.

Cooking for One: Make the whole batch, and refrigerate or freeze the leftovers in 2-cup portions.

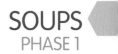

Spring Chicken Soup

Hands-On Time: 15 minutes | **Total Time:** 30 minutes | **Makes:** 4 (2¼-cup) servings

For a slightly different flavor, swap in a parsnip for the carrot here. The fresh dill gives this soup some old-fashioned flavor. For an even more flavorful soup, if you've got the time, make a batch of Homemade Chicken Broth. Simply boil together 2 bone-in skinless chicken breasts, 2 carrots, 2 small stalks celery, ½ small lemon, ½ teaspoon black peppercorns, 4 scallion greens, 2 or 3 large sprigs parsley, 2 small sprigs thyme, 1 bay leaf, 8 cups water, and ¼ teaspoon salt. Not only does this allow you to dodge the excess sodium and potential gluten that's in some canned chicken broth, you'll have cooked chicken on hand to use in salads or other dishes. Once cooled, you can freeze both the broth and chicken in whatever portion sizes you choose. Use it any time chicken broth is called for.

BELLY BUDDIES: Carrot, potatoes, green beans, bell pepper, chicken breast

- 4 cups low-sodium chicken broth (look for brands with no onions or garlic) or Homemade Chicken Broth (above)
- 2 cups water
- 1 large carrot, thinly sliced
- ½ pound small red potatoes, well scrubbed and thinly sliced

- ½ pound green beans, cut into 1-inch lengths
- 1 red bell pepper, diced
- ½ teaspoon salt
- ½ pound boneless, skinless chicken breasts, thinly sliced crosswise
- ⅔ cup frozen or fresh peas
- ½ cup chopped fresh dill

1. In a medium saucepan, bring the broth and water to a boil over medium heat. Add the carrot, potatoes, green beans, bell pepper, and salt and return to a boil. Reduce to a simmer, cover, and cook for 10 minutes, or until the potatoes are tender.

2. Add the chicken and peas and simmer, uncovered, for 2 minutes, or until the chicken is just cooked through. Stir in the dill and serve.

Per serving: 172 calories • 18g protein • 2g fat (0.5g saturated) • 5g fiber • 21g carbohydrate • 471mg sodium • 53mg magnesium

If you have gluten issues: Choose a gluten-free brand of chicken broth.

Cooking for One: Make the whole batch and refrigerate the leftovers in 2¼-cup portions. Don't freeze it, as the potatoes will get spongy.

Italian Chicken and Escarole Soup

Hands-On Time: 15 minutes | **Total Time:** 25 minutes | **Makes:** 4 (1¾-cup) servings

Choose a small, crisp head of escarole, without any tinges of yellow. The Parmesan-egg mixture added at the end makes this an Italian egg drop soup.

BELLY BUDDIES: Chicken breast, eggs

4 cups low-sodium chicken broth (look for brands with no onions or garlic) or Homemade Chicken Broth (page 111)

2 cups water

½ teaspoon dried basil

¼ teaspoon dried oregano

4 cups shredded escarole (about 4 ounces)

½ pound boneless, skinless chicken breasts, thinly sliced crosswise

2 large eggs

½ cup grated Parmesan cheese

¼ teaspoon salt

¼ teaspoon black pepper

1. In a large saucepan, combine the broth, water, basil, and oregano and bring to a boil over high heat. Reduce to a simmer, cover, and cook for 5 minutes to concentrate the flavors.

2. Add the escarole and chicken and simmer for 3 minutes.

3. Meanwhile, in a small bowl, whisk together the eggs, Parmesan, salt, and pepper.

4. Stir the egg mixture into the simmering soup and cook, stirring, for 30 seconds, or until set.

Per serving: 164 calories • 21g protein • 7g fat (3g saturated) • 1g fiber • 3g carbohydrate • 476mg sodium • 27mg magnesium

If you have gluten issues: Choose a gluten-free brand of chicken broth.

Cooking for One: Bring 1 cup broth, ½ cup water, ⅛ teaspoon dried basil, and a pinch of dried oregano to a boil and simmer for 3 minutes to concentrate the flavors. Add 1 cup shredded escarole and 2 ounces chicken breast and simmer for 2 to 3 minutes. Stir together 1 large egg, 2 tablespoons Parmesan, and a pinch each of salt and pepper. Stir it into the soup and cook for 30 seconds.

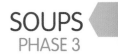

Chicken-Chard Soup with Pasta

Hands-On Time: 15 minutes | **Total Time:** 20 minutes | **Makes:** 4 (2-cup) servings

Small pasta shapes, such as anellini (which means "little rings" in Italian) or alphabet pasta, are designed to cook quickly in soups. If you have larger pasta shapes on hand, such as rigatoni or penne, cook it separately and just stir it into the soup once the chicken is cooked. Ruby chard, with its bright red stalks and crinkled leaves with touches of red, provides more than beauty to this dish. Swiss chard is a rich source of magnesium, potassium, beta-carotene and vitamins C and K. If you can't find ruby chard, green chard is fine, too.

6 cups low-sodium chicken broth (look for brands with no onions or garlic) or Homemade Chicken Broth (page 111)

2 teaspoons reduced-sodium tamari or soy sauce

2 teaspoons sesame oil

¼ teaspoon salt

¾ pound boneless, skinless chicken breast, cubed

5 cups shredded ruby chard leaves and stems (about ½ pound, or a small bunch)

¾ cup gluten-free (preferably brown rice) pastina, such as anellini or alphabets (4 ounces)

1 tablespoon rice vinegar

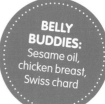

BELLY BUDDIES: Sesame oil, chicken breast, Swiss chard

1. In a large saucepan, bring the broth, tamari, sesame oil, and salt to a boil over medium-high heat.

2. Add the chicken and chard, cover, and let return to a boil. Stir in the pasta, and cook, uncovered, for 4 minutes, or until the pasta is al dente.

3. Stir in the vinegar and serve hot.

Per serving: 246 calories • 24g protein • 5g fat (1g saturated) • 4.5g fiber • 25g carbohydrate • 586mg sodium • 95mg magnesium

If you have gluten issues: Choose gluten-free brands of chicken broth and tamari.

Cooking for One: Make the whole soup, but do not add the pasta. Cook the chicken and chard for only 2 minutes and add the vinegar. Divide the soup into 4 equal portions, and refrigerate or freeze. For each portion of soup, bring to a boil in a small saucepan, add 3 tablespoons pastina, and cook for 4 minutes, or until al dente.

Mexican Spinach and Chicken Soup

Hands-On Time: 20 minutes | **Total Time:** 30 minutes | **Makes:** 4 (2¼-cup) servings

Both the leaves and the stems of cilantro are packed with flavor, so use both here. If you've got leftover cilantro, wrap it in dampened paper towels, place in a plastic bag, and refrigerate. It'll keep for several days.

BELLY BUDDIES: Olive oil, spinach, sesame seeds, chicken breast, lime

- 1 tablespoon extra-virgin olive oil
- 1½ teaspoons ground coriander
- 1½ teaspoons ground cumin
- 4 cups low-sodium chicken broth (look for brands with no onions or garlic) or Homemade Chicken Broth (page 111)
- ½ teaspoon salt
- 1¼ cups water

- 1 package (10 ounces) frozen chopped spinach, thawed (no need to squeeze dry)
- 2 tablespoons cornmeal
- 1 tablespoon sesame seeds
- ½ pound boneless, skinless chicken breast, cut crosswise into ¼-inch-thick slices
- ¾ cup cilantro leaves and stems, finely chopped
- 2 tablespoons fresh lime juice

1. In a Dutch oven or 5-quart saucepan, heat the oil over medium heat. Add the coriander and cumin and cook for 1 minute to toast the spices.

2. Add the broth, salt, and 1 cup of the water and bring to a boil. Reduce to a simmer, cover, and cook for 5 minutes to concentrate the flavors.

3. Add the spinach and simmer, uncovered, for 2 minutes, or until the spinach is heated through.

4. In a small bowl, combine the cornmeal, sesame seeds, and the remaining ¼ cup water. Stir the mixture into the soup along with the chicken and cook for 2 to 3 minutes, or until the chicken is cooked through and the soup is lightly thickened. Stir in the cilantro and lime juice and serve.

Per serving: 171 calories • 18g protein • 7g fat (1g saturated) • 3g fiber • 9g carbohydrate • 483mg sodium • 79mg magnesium

If you have gluten issues: Choose a gluten-free brand of chicken broth.

Cooking for One: Make the whole batch, and refrigerate or freeze the leftovers in 2¼-cup portions.

Italian Tomato and Meatball Soup

Hands-On Time: 20 minutes | **Total Time:** 40 minutes | **Makes:** 4 (2-cup) servings

Since you may need to buy a full pound of turkey to get what you need for this recipe, go ahead and make a double batch of meatballs. Then save half (in the fridge or freezer) to toss into a simmering tomato sauce for spaghetti and meatballs. Kale is one of our favorite low-FODMAP superfoods—it's rich in beta-carotene and vitamins C and K.

½ pound 93% lean ground turkey

4 ounces Italian turkey sausage, crumbled (look for brands with no onions or garlic)

2 tablespoons oat bran

1 tablespoon chia seeds

1 large egg white

4 cups low-sodium chicken broth (look for brands with no onions or garlic) or Homemade Chicken Broth (page 111).

2 cups water

1 can (14.5 ounces) no-salt-added fire-roasted diced tomatoes (look for brands with no onions or garlic)

¼ teaspoon salt

4 cups shredded kale (about 4 ounces)

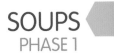

BELLY BUDDIES: Lean turkey, oats, chia seeds, egg, tomatoes, kale

1. In a small bowl, combine the ground turkey, sausage, oat bran, chia seeds, and egg white and mix until well combined. Shape into 12 meatballs.

2. In a large saucepan, bring the broth, water, tomatoes, and salt to a boil over high heat. Reduce to a simmer and add the kale and meatballs. Cover and simmer for 10 minutes, or until the meatballs are cooked through.

Per serving: 215 calories • 25g protein • 7g fat (2g saturated) • 3.5g fiber • 17g carbohydrate • 492mg sodium • 48mg magnesium

If you have gluten issues: Choose gluten-free brands of sausage, oat bran, chia seeds, and chicken broth.

Butternut Squash, Turkey, and Red Quinoa Soup

Hands-On Time: 15 minutes | **Total Time:** 35 minutes | **Makes:** 4 (1½-cup) servings

Carrot juice can be found with refrigerated juices but also comes in shelf-stable form, in bottles. If you can't find it, make this with low-sodium mixed vegetable juice instead. Lutein, a carotenoid found in carrots, lowers the risk of colon cancer.

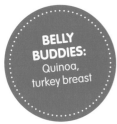

BELLY BUDDIES: Quinoa, turkey breast

½ cup red quinoa

Water

1 tablespoon plus 1 teaspoon extra-virgin olive oil

1 teaspoon curry powder (look for brands with no onions or garlic)

½ pound turkey breast cutlets (steaks), cut into ½-inch chunks

2 cups low-sodium chicken broth (look for brands with no onions or garlic)

1 cup carrot juice

1½ cups water

2 teaspoons grated lemon zest

½ teaspoon salt

¼ teaspoon black pepper

½ pound butternut squash, cut into cubes (⅓-inch)

Lemon wedges

1. Soak the quinoa in a bowl of water to cover while you begin the soup.

2. In a medium nonstick saucepan, heat the oil and curry powder over medium-high heat. Add the turkey and cook for 1 to 2 minutes, or until opaque all over but still pink on the inside (it cooks more later). With a slotted spoon, transfer the turkey to a bowl.

3. Add the broth, carrot juice, water, lemon zest, salt, and pepper and bring to a simmer. Drain the quinoa and add to the soup. Bring to a boil, then reduce to a simmer, cover tightly, and cook for 5 minutes.

4. Add the squash and bring back to a simmer. Cover and cook for 15 minutes, or until the quinoa is tender.

5. Stir in the turkey (and any juices) and cook for 2 minutes to finish cooking. Serve the soup with lemon wedges for squeezing.

Per serving: 239 calories • 19g protein • 6g fat (0.5g saturated) • 3g fiber • 28g carbohydrate • 422mg sodium • 29mg magnesium

If you have gluten issues: Choose gluten-free brands of curry powder and chicken broth.

Cooking for One: Make the whole batch, and refrigerate or freeze the leftovers in 1½-cup portions.

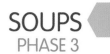

Turkey Soup with Multigrain Dumplings

Hands-On Time: 25 minutes | **Total Time:** 35 minutes | **Makes:** 4 (1½-cup) servings

You can also have this soup on Phases 1 and 2 if you leave out the dumplings. Divide the soup into three 2-cup portions and top each serving with 1 tablespoon grated Parmesan cheese.

DUMPLINGS

- ⅔ cup brown rice flour
- ⅓ cup almond flour
- 3 tablespoons ground flaxseed
- 1½ teaspoons baking powder
- 1 teaspoon chia seeds
- ¼ teaspoon salt
- 2 tablespoons snipped chives or sliced scallion greens
- 1 large egg
- 2 tablespoons water

SOUP

- 2 teaspoons extra-virgin olive oil
- 2 carrots, diced
- 1 green bell pepper, diced
- 2 teaspoons grated lemon zest
- ½ teaspoon dried thyme
- ¼ teaspoon salt
- ¼ teaspoon black pepper
- 10 ounces ground turkey breast
- 5 cups low-sodium chicken broth (look for brands with no onions or garlic)

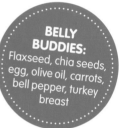

BELLY BUDDIES: Flaxseed, chia seeds, egg, olive oil, carrots, bell pepper, turkey breast

1. **Prepare the dumplings:** In a medium bowl, combine the rice and almond flours, flaxseeds, baking powder, chia seeds, and salt and blend well. Stir in the chives. Make a well in the center and break in the egg. Add the water. Blend into the flour mixture. Divide the dough into 12 equal portions and roll into balls.

2. **Make the soup:** In a large nonstick saucepan or Dutch oven, heat the oil over medium-high heat. Add the carrots, bell pepper, lemon zest, thyme, salt, and pepper and cook for 1 minute. Add the turkey and break it into fine crumbles.

3. Add the broth, cover, and bring to a gentle simmer over medium-high heat. Add the dumplings. When they rise to the surface, cover, and very gently simmer for 10 minutes, or until cooked through.

4. Serve 3 dumplings per person.

Per serving: 330 calories • 28g protein • 12g fat (1g saturated) • 5g fiber • 32g carbohydrate • 593mg sodium • 39mg magnesium

If you have gluten issues: Choose gluten-free brands of baking powder, chia seeds, and chicken broth.

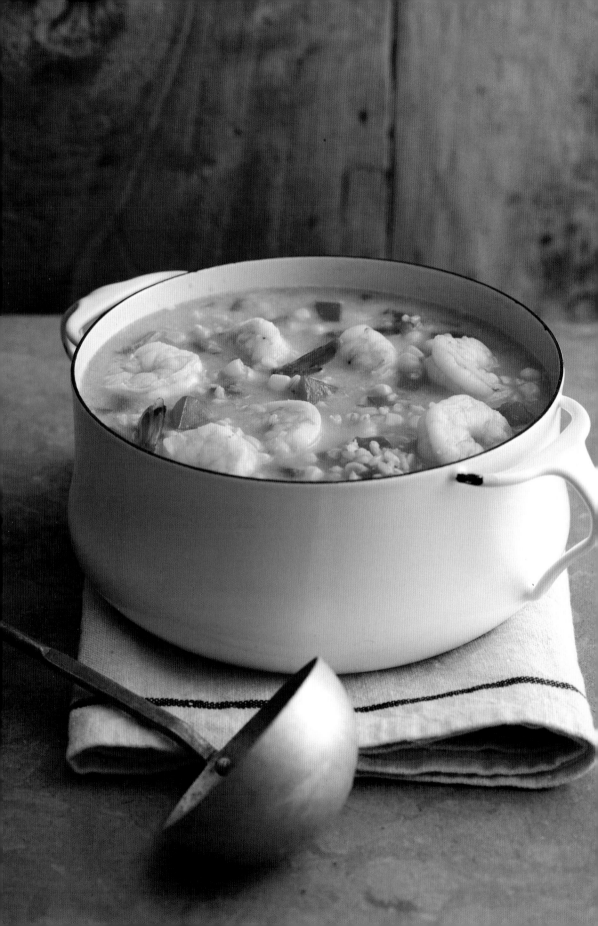

Coconut Shrimp Soup

Hands-On Time: 25 minutes | **Total Time:** 40 minutes | **Makes:** 4 (1¼-cup) servings

Roasted Garlic Oil (page 54) is used in this soup to lend a slightly nutty garlic flavor, but feel free to swap in extra-virgin olive oil for the garlic oil, if you'd prefer.

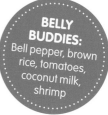

BELLY BUDDIES: Bell pepper, brown rice, tomatoes, coconut milk, shrimp

1 tablespoon Roasted Garlic Oil (page 54)

1 red bell pepper, diced

¼ cup quick-cooking brown rice

½ pound plum tomatoes, diced

1½ cups water

½ teaspoon salt

¼ teaspoon red-pepper flakes

1 cup light coconut milk

¾ pound large shrimp, peeled, deveined, and halved horizontally

1 cup frozen corn kernels, thawed

1 tablespoon fresh lime juice

1. In a medium saucepan, heat the oil over medium heat. Add the bell pepper and cook, stirring occasionally, for 5 minutes, or until crisp-tender. Add the rice, stir to coat, and cook for 1 minute.

2. Add the tomatoes, water, salt, and pepper flakes and bring to a boil. Reduce to a simmer, cover, and cook for 10 minutes, or until the rice is tender.

3. Add the coconut milk, shrimp, and corn and simmer, uncovered until the shrimp are just cooked through, about 1 minute. Remove from the heat and stir in the lime juice.

Per serving: 240 calories • 19g protein • 8.5g fat (3g saturated) • 3g fiber • 24g carbohydrate • 497mg sodium • 38mg magnesium

Provençal Fish Soup

Hands-On Time: 30 minutes | **Total Time:** 40 minutes | **Makes:** 4 (generous 1½-cup) servings

Fresh fennel, sometimes called anise, has a mild licorice flavor and a texture similar to celery. If you're not a big fan of the anise flavor, you can swap in 2 stalks of celery for the fresh fennel and omit the fennel seeds.

BELLY BUDDIES: Olive oil, carrot, tomatoes, potatoes, cod

1 tablespoon plus 1 teaspoon extra-virgin olive oil

1 bulb fennel (about 1 pound), stalks discarded, thinly sliced

1 large carrot, thinly sliced

1 teaspoon fennel seeds

4 cups water

1 can (14.5 ounces) no-salt-added fire-roasted diced tomatoes (look for brands with no onions or garlic)

2 strips orange zest (2 x ½ inches each)

¾ teaspoon salt

½ pound russet (baking) potatoes, peeled and thinly sliced

½ pound skinless cod fillets, cut into 1-inch chunks

1. In a large saucepan, heat the oil over medium heat. Add the fennel bulb, carrot, and fennel seeds and cook, stirring occasionally, for 7 minutes, or until the fennel bulb is golden and both the fennel and carrot are crisp-tender.

2. Add the water, tomatoes, orange zest, and salt and bring to a boil. Cook for 5 minutes to concentrate the flavors.

3. Add the potatoes, reduce to a simmer, cover, and cook for 10 minutes, or until the potatoes are tender.

4. Add the cod, cover, and cook for 5 minutes, or until just cooked through.

Per serving: 196 calories • 14g protein • 5.5g fat (0.5g saturated) • 6g fiber • 25g carbohydrate • 552mg sodium • 52mg magnesium

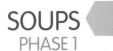

Fennel-Potato Soup

Hands-On Time: 10 minutes | **Total Time:** 25 minutes | **Makes:** 4 (1½-cup) servings

The potatoes for this soup are purposely cut into two different sizes. The larger size will maintain its shape, and the smaller size will break down as the soup cooks, helping to give the soup a little heft. If the fennel you buy has the feathery fronds attached, set some aside to garnish the soup.

- 1 tablespoon plus 1 teaspoon extra-virgin olive oil
- 1 large bulb fennel, stalks discarded, cored and diced
- ¼ cup water
- 1 pound russet (baking) potatoes, well scrubbed, half cut into ½-inch cubes, half cut into ¼-inch dice
- 3 cups low-sodium chicken broth (look for brands with no onions or garlic)

- 2 teaspoons hot paprika
- ¼ teaspoon salt
- ¼ teaspoon black pepper
- ⅓ cup chopped fresh cilantro
- ¾ cup crumbled reduced-fat feta cheese (3 ounces)
- 4 teaspoons hulled sunflower seeds

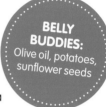

BELLY BUDDIES: Olive oil, potatoes, sunflower seeds

1. In a medium-large saucepan, heat the oil over medium-high heat. Add the fennel and toss to coat. Reduce the heat to medium, add the water, cover, and cook, stirring once or twice, for 8 minutes, or until the fennel is tender and begins to sizzle in the oil.

2. Stir in the potatoes, broth, paprika, salt, and pepper. Cover and bring to a boil. Reduce to a simmer and cook for 8 minutes, or until the larger pieces of potato are tender.

3. Stir in the cilantro. Top each serving of soup with 3 tablespoons feta and 1 teaspoon sunflower seeds.

Per serving: 227 calories • 10g protein • 9g fat (2.5g saturated) • 4.5g fiber • 29g carbohydrate • 541mg sodium • 50mg magnesium

If you have gluten issues: Choose gluten-free brands of chicken broth and paprika.

Rich Carrot and Chickpea Soup

Hands-On Time: 10 minutes | **Total Time:** 25 minutes | **Makes:** 4 (1½-cup) servings

Peanut butter adds a toasty richness to soups. But it's not just about flavor—peanut butter also adds healthy fats, a modest amount of protein, and magnesium. We like all-natural peanut butter made without added sugar and artery-clogging fats. If you prefer a chunkier texture, in step 4, puree about half the carrots before stirring in the chickpeas.

BELLY BUDDIES: Olive oil, carrots, peanut butter

- 1 tablespoon Roasted Garlic Oil (page 54) or extra-virgin olive oil
- 1 pound carrots, cut into ⅓-inch dice
- ¼ cup no-salt-added tomato paste (look for brands with no onions or garlic)
- 1 teaspoon ground coriander
- ¾ teaspoon salt
- 4 cups water
- 3 tablespoons natural peanut butter
- 1 cup canned no-salt-added chickpeas, rinsed and drained
- Parsley or cilantro leaves and cracked black pepper (optional)

1. In a nonstick soup pot or Dutch oven, heat the oil over medium-high heat. Add the carrots and stir to coat with the oil.

2. Stir in the tomato paste, coriander, salt, and water and stir to make a broth. Bring to a boil, then reduce to a simmer, partially cover, and cook for 7 minutes, or until the carrots are crisp-tender.

3. In a small bowl, stir a little bit of the hot soup broth into the peanut butter to loosen it up. Stir the mixture into the soup.

4. Stir in the chickpeas. With an immersion blender (or in a standard blender), puree until smooth.

5. Serve hot, garnished with parsley and pepper, if desired.

Per serving: 231 calories • 8g protein • 10g fat (1.5g saturated) • 7.5g fiber • 28g carbohydrate • 539mg sodium • 41mg magnesium

Cooking for One: Make the whole batch, and refrigerate or freeze the leftovers in 1½-cup portions.

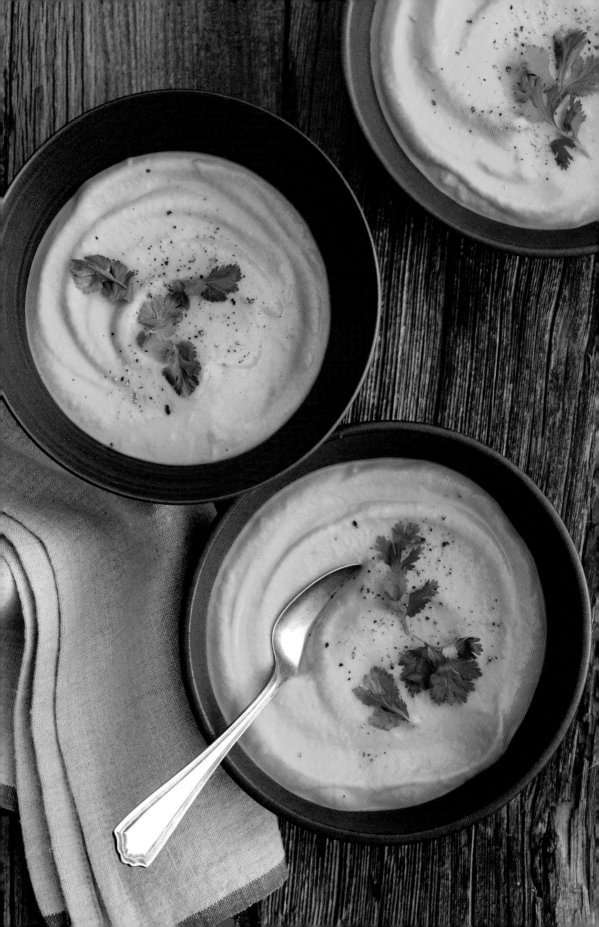

Kale and Basmati Soup with Pumpkin Seed Pesto

Hands-On Time: 10 minutes | **Total Time:** 30 minutes | **Makes:** 4 (2-cup) servings

The quick-cooking rice breaks up as the soup cooks and helps create a thick, creamy texture. Be sure to stir the pesto into the soup well, to make it creamy and give it a good flavor boost. In addition to magnesium, pumpkin seeds are rich in manganese, an important nutrient that plays a role in blood sugar management.

BELLY BUDDIES: Brown rice, carrots, kale, pumpkin seeds, lemon

- 5 cups low-sodium chicken broth (look for brands with no onions or garlic)
- ½ teaspoon salt
- ¼ teaspoon black pepper
- ¼ teaspoon grated nutmeg
- 2¼ cups water
- ½ cup quick-cooking brown basmati rice
- 4 large carrots, halved lengthwise and thinly sliced crosswise
- 1 package (16 ounces) frozen chopped kale, thawed
- ¼ cup hulled pumpkin seeds (pepitas), toasted
- ½ cup packed fresh basil leaves
- ¼ cup grated Parmesan cheese
- 2 tablespoons fresh lemon juice

1. In a large saucepan, combine the broth, salt, pepper, nutmeg, and 2 cups of the water and bring to a boil over high heat. Add the rice, carrots, and kale and return to a boil. Reduce to a simmer, cover, and cook for 20 minutes, or until the rice and kale are very tender.

2. Meanwhile, in a small heavy skillet, heat the pumpkin seeds for 2 minutes, or until they begin to pop. Transfer to a mini food processor and add the basil, cheese, and the remaining ¼ cup water. Puree until smooth. Scrape the pesto into a small bowl.

3. Stir the lemon juice into the soup. Each serving of soup gets 2 tablespoons pesto that should be stirred in before eating.

Per serving: 222 calories • 12g protein • 6.5g fat (2g saturated) • 5g fiber • 31g carbohydrate • 519mg sodium • 105mg magnesium

If you have gluten issues: Choose a gluten-free brand of chicken broth.

Cooking for One: Make the whole batch, and refrigerate or freeze the leftovers in 2-cup portions. The pesto can also be refrigerated or frozen; divide it into 2-tablespoon chunks before freezing.

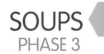

Spiced Tofu and Vegetable Soup

Hands-On Time: 25 minutes | **Total Time:** 40 minutes | **Makes:** 4 (3-cup) servings

Sesame oil, added at the end of the cooking time, gives this soup a robust, slightly smoky flavor. Once opened, the sesame oil should be stored in the refrigerator where it will keep up to 1 year.

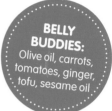

BELLY BUDDIES: Olive oil, carrots, tomatoes, ginger, tofu, sesame oil

- 2 teaspoons extra-virgin olive oil
- 2 medium carrots, shredded with a vegetable peeler
- ½ pound plum tomatoes, coarsely chopped (1 cup)
- 1 piece (3 inches) fresh ginger, peeled and cut into matchsticks
- ¼ teaspoon red-pepper flakes
- 6 cups water
- ½ teaspoon salt

- 1 can (15 ounces) baby corn, drained and rinsed
- 1 can (8 ounces) sliced bamboo shoots, drained and rinsed
- 15 snow peas (about ¼ pound), cut crosswise into bite-size pieces
- 1 container (14 ounces) extra-firm tofu, drained and cut into 1-inch chunks
- 1 tablespoon rice vinegar
- 2 teaspoons sesame oil

1. In a large saucepan, heat the olive oil over medium heat. Add the carrots, tomatoes, and ginger and cook, stirring occasionally, for 5 minutes, or until the carrots have started to soften. Stir in the pepper flakes.

2. Add the water and salt and bring to a boil. Stir in the corn and bamboo shoots and boil for 5 minutes to concentrate the flavors.

3. Reduce to a simmer, add the snow peas and tofu, and cook for 2 minutes, or until the snow peas are bright green and the tofu is heated through. Stir in the rice vinegar and sesame oil and serve.

Per serving: 286 calories • 16g protein • 12g fat (1.5g saturated) • 7g fiber • 34g carbohydrate • 593mg sodium • 48mg magnesium

Cooking for One: Make the whole batch and refrigerate the leftovers in 3-cup portions.

Hazelnut-Stuffed Pork Chops

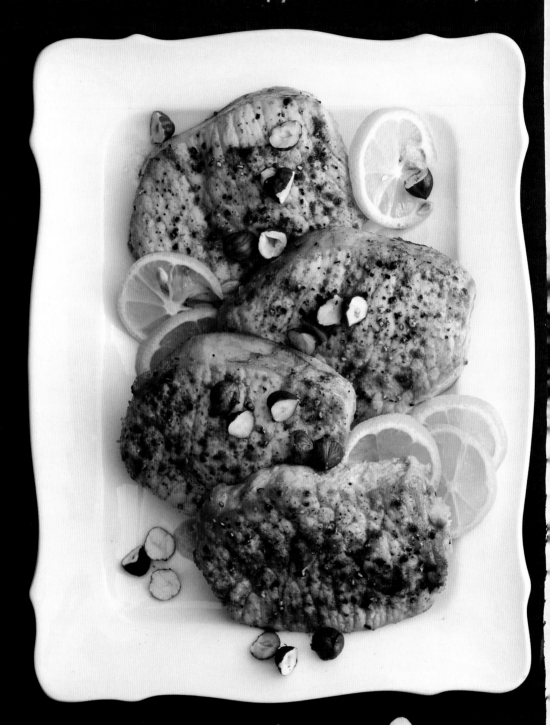

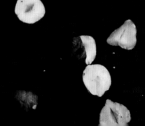

Rich in anti-inflammatory fats

Chapter 6

★ MAIN ★ COURSES

Beloved mealtime favorites

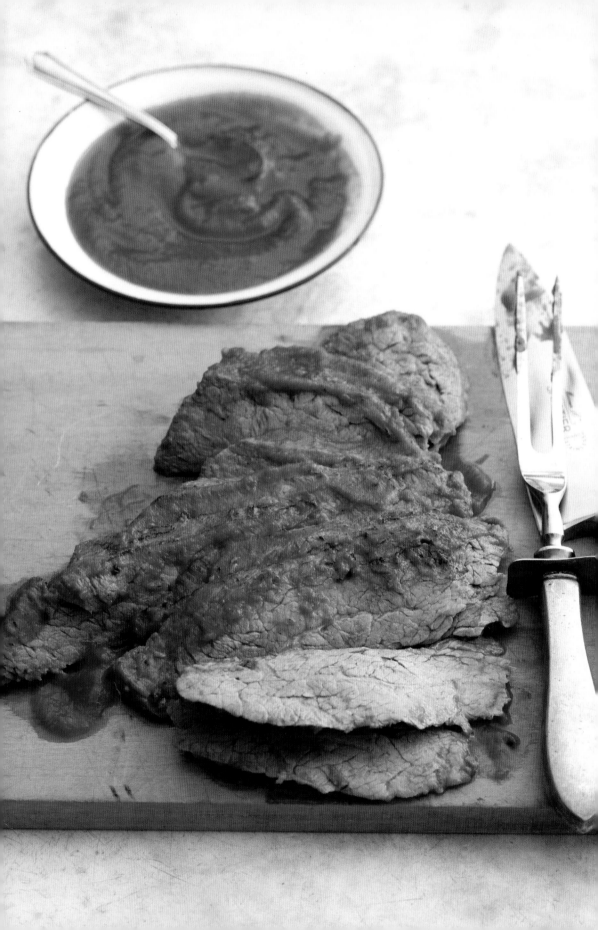

Barbecue-Glazed Flank Steak

Hands-On Time: 20 minutes | **Total Time:** 45 minutes | **Makes:** 4 servings

The best way to ensure that the barbecue sauce you're using doesn't have onion, garlic, or notoriously unhealthy high-fructose corn syrup in it is to make your own. You can make the sauce well ahead and store it in the refrigerator until you're ready to broil the steak. You can also make it in a larger batch. Just double all the ingredients and cook until it's reduced to 2 cups; the cooking time should be about the same.

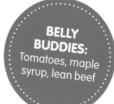

BELLY BUDDIES: Tomatoes, maple syrup, lean beef

- 1 can (15 ounces) no-salt-added crushed tomatoes (look for brands with no onions or garlic)
- 2 tablespoons pure maple syrup
- 2 tablespoons balsamic, red wine, or distilled apple cider vinegar
- 1 teaspoon smoked paprika
- ¾ teaspoon salt
- ½ teaspoon chipotle chile powder or mild chili powder blend (look for brands with no onions or garlic)
- ½ teaspoon ground cumin
- 1 pound flank steak

1. Preheat the broiler with a rack 6 inches from the heat. Line a baking sheet with foil and place a wire cooling rack on the baking sheet.

2. In a blender or mini food processor, combine the tomatoes, maple syrup, vinegar, paprika, salt, chile powder, and cumin. Process to a smooth puree.

3. Transfer to a small saucepan and bring to a simmer over medium heat. Reduce to medium-low and simmer, stirring often (use a splatter screen if you have one), for 15 minutes, or until the sauce is thickened and reduced to a generous 1 cup. Measure out ⅓ cup of the sauce to use for basting. Set the remainder aside for serving.

4. Place the flank steak on the wire rack and baste with half the sauce. Broil for 6 minutes. Flip the steak over and brush with half the remaining sauce. Broil for 3 minutes. Brush with the remaining sauce and broil until the steak is cooked to your desired doneness, 3 to 6 minutes for medium-rare (depending on the thickness of the steak).

5. Let the steak rest for 10 minutes before thinly slicing across the grain. Serve with the reserved sauce spooned on top.

Per serving: 225 calories • 26g protein • 6.5g fat (2.5g saturated) • 2g fiber • 12g carbohydrate • 506mg sodium • 57mg magnesium

If you have gluten issues: Choose a gluten-free brand of paprika.

Tex-Mex Cheeseburgers

Hands-On Time: 20 minutes | **Total Time:** 20 minutes | **Makes:** 4 servings

If you have trouble finding ground sirloin, try this with 95% extra lean ground beef. Pickled jalapeño peppers—both whole and sliced—are predictably hot, unlike their fresh counterparts, which can vary from mild to blazing. For a milder burger (although these aren't too spicy), scrape the seeds out of the jalapeño before chopping. Serve with Pickled Zucchini Spears (page 240).

BELLY BUDDIES: Lean beef, avocado, tomato

- 1 pound ground sirloin
- 2 tablespoons no-salt-added tomato paste (look for brands with no onions or garlic)
- 1 pickled jalapeño chile pepper, finely chopped
- ½ teaspoon salt
- ¼ teaspoon black pepper
- 2 ounces sliced reduced-fat Monterey jack cheese
- ½ avocado, mashed
- 1 beefsteak tomato, thickly sliced

1. Preheat the broiler with the rack 4 inches from the heat.

2. In a large bowl, combine the beef, tomato paste, chile pepper, salt, and black pepper. Shape into four 4-inch-wide patties. Place on the broiler pan and broil for 2 minutes per side for medium; 1½ minutes per side for rare; or 3 minutes per side for well-done.

3. Divide the cheese slices among the burgers. Broil for 1 minute, or until the cheese melts. Top with mashed avocado (about 2 tablespoons per burger) and a tomato slice.

Per serving: 245 calories • 25g protein • 14g fat (5g saturated) • 2g fiber • 6g carbohydrate • 528mg sodium • 14mg magnesium

Cooking for One: Combine ¼ pound ground sirloin with 1½ teaspoons tomato paste, ½ teaspoon chopped jalapeño, ⅛ teaspoon salt, and a pinch of black pepper. Shape and broil as directed. Top with ½ ounce reduced-fat Monterey jack cheese and broil for 1 minute, or until the cheese melts. Top with 2 tablespoons mashed avocado and a slice of tomato.

Egg-Stuffed Meat Loaf

Hands-On Time: 25 minutes | **Total Time:** 55 minutes | **Makes:** 4 servings

Rolled oats take the place of bread crumbs in this loaf, while shredded potatoes supply moisture. When the loaf is sliced, the eggs hidden inside are revealed. Serve with Arugula Salad with Pine Nuts and Parmesan (page 214) and steamed carrots. Beef is a rich source of heme iron, a highly absorbable form of this mineral that helps transport oxygen throughout our bodies.

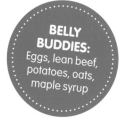

2 large eggs

1 pound ground sirloin

1 russet (baking) potato (8 ounces), peeled and shredded

¼ cup rolled oats

2 tablespoons lactose-free 1% milk

¼ cup chopped fresh parsley

¾ teaspoon dried thyme

½ teaspoon salt

½ teaspoon black pepper

2 teaspoons Dijon mustard (look for brands with no onions or garlic)

1½ teaspoons pure maple syrup

BELLY BUDDIES: Eggs, lean beef, potatoes, oats, maple syrup

1. Place the eggs in a small saucepan with water to cover. Bring to a boil over high heat, then remove from the heat, cover, and let stand for 12 minutes. Drain, run under cold water, crack, and peel.

2. Preheat the oven to 375°F.

3. In a large bowl, combine the ground beef, potato, oats, milk, parsley, thyme, salt, and pepper.

4. Shape half of the mixture into a 6 x 3-inch rectangle on a small rimmed baking sheet and make a trench down the center. Place the eggs, lengthwise and touching, in the trench. Top with the remaining meat mixture, pressing it firmly to enclose the eggs.

5. In a small bowl, stir together the mustard and maple syrup and brush it on the top of the loaf. Bake for 30 minutes, or until set and cooked through. Divide the loaf into 4 equal slices and serve 1 slice per person.

Per serving: 244 calories • 27g protein • 8g fat (3g saturated) • 1.5g fiber • 17g carbohydrate • 460mg sodium • 20mg magnesium

If you have gluten issues: Choose gluten-free brands of oats and mustard.

Cooking for One: Omit the eggs, but otherwise, bake the entire meat loaf as directed. Divide the loaf into 4 equal slices. Eat one now and refrigerate or freeze the remaining slices. Refrigerated slices will keep up to 5 days, frozen up to 3 months.

Hazelnut-Stuffed Pork Chops

Hands-On Time: 10 minutes | **Total Time:** 25 minutes | **Makes:** 4 servings

You can switch out the hazelnuts for another nut, such as almonds or pecans, or try the stuffing with pumpkin seeds or sunflower seeds. Hazelnuts provide a nice dose of magnesium, which keeps inflammation at bay. Serve the chops with Crispy-Topped Broiled Tomatoes (page 243) and steamed broccoli.

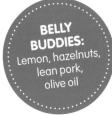

BELLY BUDDIES:
Lemon, hazelnuts, lean pork, olive oil

1 lemon

¼ cup blanched hazelnuts

½ teaspoon paprika

⅛ teaspoon salt

4 thick-cut (¾ to 1 inch) boneless pork loin chops (4 ounces each)

2 teaspoons extra-virgin olive oil

½ teaspoon ground cumin

¼ teaspoon black pepper

1. Preheat the oven to 375°F. Line a baking sheet with foil (for easier cleanup).

2. Grate 1 teaspoon of lemon zest and set aside. Halve the lemon and squeeze 1 tablespoon juice and set aside. Reserve both lemon halves.

3. In a mini food processor, process the hazelnuts until coarsely ground. Pulse in the lemon zest, paprika, and salt. Add the reserved lemon juice and process until a thick paste forms.

4. With a sharp knife, make a horizontal pocket in the pork chops. Stuff each chop with a tablespoon of the hazelnut mixture, pressing it thin. Press the open edges of the pork together.

5. Rub the pork with the oil. Season with the cumin and pepper. Place the pork on the baking sheet and bake for 10 minutes. Then turn the chops over and bake for 3 to 5 minutes longer (depending on the thickness), or until cooked through but still juicy.

6. Squeeze the reserved lemon halves over the pork and serve hot.

Per serving: 233 calories • 23g protein • 15g fat (3g saturated) • 1g fiber • 3g carbohydrate • 120mg sodium • 36mg magnesium

If you have gluten issues: Choose a gluten-free brand of paprika.

Cooking for One: Make the full amount of filling and save the extra to (1) stuff more pork chops, (2) stuff boneless chicken breasts, or (3) use as a savory spread for a snack. Stuff 1 pork chop and bake as directed (baking times are the same).

Maple-Rosemary Roasted Pork Tenderloin

Hands-On Time: 10 minutes | **Total Time:** 40 minutes | **Makes:** 4 servings

Maple syrup is easier on digestion than table sugar, due to its lower fructose content, and it pairs nicely with pungent rosemary. For the best, most robust maple flavor, look for grade B maple syrup. Serve the pork with Home Fries (page 256) and steamed broccoli.

- 1 pound pork tenderloin
- ¾ teaspoon crumbled dried rosemary
- ¾ teaspoon coarse (kosher) salt
- ½ teaspoon black pepper
- 3 teaspoons extra-virgin olive oil
- 1 tablespoon plus 1 teaspoon pure maple syrup
- 1 teaspoon distilled apple cider vinegar
- ¾ teaspoon Dijon mustard (look for brands with no onions or garlic)

BELLY BUDDIES: Lean pork, olive oil, maple syrup

1. Preheat the oven to 375°F.

2. Place the pork in a small roasting pan and sprinkle the rosemary, salt, and pepper over the top, rubbing them into the pork. Brush with 2 teaspoons of the oil. Roast for 20 minutes.

3. Meanwhile, in a small bowl, combine the maple syrup, vinegar, mustard, and the remaining 1 teaspoon oil.

4. After the pork has cooked for 20 minutes, brush it with the maple syrup mixture. Roast for 10 minutes longer, or until just cooked through but still juicy, and an instant-read thermometer registers 145°F.

Per serving: 174 calories • 24g protein • 6g fat (1.5g saturated) • 0g fiber • 5g carbohydrate • 444mg sodium • 33mg magnesium

If you have gluten issues: Choose a gluten-free brand of mustard.

Cooking for One: The leftover pork makes great lunches, but if 1 pound seems like a lot to consume, you can make a half recipe. Sprinkle a ½-pound piece of pork tenderloin with ½ teaspoon each rosemary and salt and ¼ teaspoon pepper, and brush with 1 teaspoon oil. Roast for 20 minutes. Combine 2 teaspoons maple syrup, and ½ teaspoon each vinegar, mustard, and oil. Brush on the pork and roast until just cooked through. Have half for dinner and save the remainder for a lunch or dinner salad.

Seared Pork Chops with Pineapple Sauce

Hands-On Time: 15 minutes | **Total Time:** 20 minutes | **Makes:** 4 servings

If you like, pick up some cut-up fresh pineapple from the produce department or salad bar. Finely chop it and use it in place of the canned crushed pineapple. Serve the pork with Zesty Orange and White Potato Salad (page 227) and steamed green beans.

BELLY BUDDIES:
Olive oil, lean pork, pineapple

1 tablespoon Roasted Garlic Oil (page 54) or extra-virgin olive oil

¾ teaspoon coarse (kosher) salt

4 boneless pork loin chops (4 ounces each)

¼ cup sliced scallion greens or snipped chives

1 can (8 ounces) juice-packed crushed pineapple, drained

½ cup low-sodium chicken broth (look for brands with no onions or garlic) or Homemade Chicken Broth (page 111)

¼ teaspoon dried thyme

⅛ teaspoon cayenne pepper

1. In a large nonstick skillet, heat the oil over medium heat. Sprinkle ½ teaspoon of the salt over the pork. Add the pork to the skillet and cook for 1½ minutes per side, or until lightly browned and just cooked through.

2. Remove the pork and set aside. Add the scallion greens to the skillet and cook for 1 minute, or until softened. Add the pineapple, broth, thyme, cayenne, and remaining ¼ teaspoon salt. Bring to a boil and cook for 2 minutes, or until the liquid has almost evaporated.

3. To serve, spoon the sauce (about ¼ cup) over each pork chop.

Per serving: 246 calories • 24g protein • 12g fat (4g saturated) • 0.5g fiber • 9g carbohydrate • 404mg sodium • 26mg magnesium

If you have gluten issues: Choose a gluten-free brand of chicken broth.

Chicken-Fried Pork with Fresh Tomato Relish

Hands-On Time: 30 minutes | **Total Time:** 30 minutes | **Makes:** 4 servings

Pork turns out incredibly moist and tender when cooked in a blanket of egg and cornstarch. Tenderloin is one of the leanest cuts, with all the flavor but little fat. Serve with steamed spinach and Maple-Glazed Carrots (page 250).

½ pound beefsteak tomatoes, diced

⅓ cup fresh parsley, chopped

1 tablespoon snipped fresh chives or sliced scallion greens

1 tablespoon red wine vinegar

½ teaspoon salt

½ teaspoon black pepper

¾ pound pork tenderloin, cut crosswise into 4 pieces

2 tablespoons potato starch

1 large egg white

2 tablespoons extra-virgin olive oil

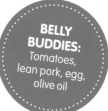

BELLY BUDDIES: Tomatoes, lean pork, egg, olive oil

1. In a medium bowl, stir together the tomatoes, parsley, chives, vinegar, salt, and pepper.

2. Place a piece of pork on a work surface and make a horizontal cut almost, but not quite, through it, then open the way you would the page of a book. Flatten slightly by pressing down on the pork with your hands. Repeat for all the pork.

3. Place the potato starch in one bowl. In a separate bowl, beat the egg white with 2 teaspoons of water to combine. Dip the pork in the potato starch and then in the egg white mixture. In a large nonstick skillet, heat 1 tablespoon of the oil over medium-high heat. Add half the pork and cook for 3 minutes per side, or until golden brown and cooked through. Repeat with the remaining oil and pork.

4. Serve the pork topped with the tomato relish.

Per serving: 186 calories • 19g protein • 9g fat (1.5g saturated) • 1g fiber • 6g carbohydrate • 356mg sodium • 34mg magnesium

Grilled Chicken with Salsa Verde

Hands-On Time: 5 minutes | **Total Time:** 15 minutes plus standing time | **Makes:** 4 servings

Serve the chicken with boiled new potatoes and grilled zucchini or eggplant. If you're on Phase 3, serve it alongside Sunny Kasha (page 260). While you've got the grill going, cook up a couple of extra chicken breasts for the upcoming week. The cooked chicken should keep at least 3 days in the refrigerator (store it in an airtight container in a single layer), so don't grill more than you can eat within the week. Experiment with different rubs, using about ¼ teaspoon of rub per chicken breast. Try one of the spice blends in Chapter 2.

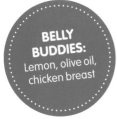

BELLY BUDDIES:
Lemon, olive oil, chicken breast

- 1 cup packed fresh flat-leaf parsley leaves
- ¼ cup water
- 1 tablespoon lemon juice
- 2 teaspoons extra-virgin olive oil
- ½ teaspoon salt
- ½ teaspoon curry powder (look for brands with no onions or garlic)
- ½ teaspoon ground coriander
- 4 boneless, skinless chicken breast halves (6 ounces each)

1. In a mini food processor, combine the parsley, water, lemon juice, oil, and ¼ teaspoon of the salt. Process to a smooth puree.

2. Preheat the grill or a grill pan to medium-high. Rub the grill rack or pan with a little oil.

3. In a small bowl, combine the curry powder, coriander, and the remaining ¼ teaspoon salt.

4. Rub the chicken all over with the spice mixture and grill for 4 to 6 minutes per side, or until cooked through but still faintly pink in the center. Let stand for 5 minutes before serving.

5. Serve the chicken with the parsley sauce spooned on top.

Per serving: 222 calories • 37g protein • 7g fat (1.5g saturated) • 0.5g fiber • 2g carbohydrate • 497mg sodium • 53mg magnesium

If you have gluten issues: Choose a gluten-free brand of curry powder.

Cooking for One: Rub 1 chicken breast half all over with a mixture of ⅛ teaspoon each curry powder and coriander. Sprinkle with a pinch of salt. Grill as directed. Make the full amount of parsley sauce and use 1½ tablespoons per serving. The extra sauce will keep in the fridge for 2 weeks. Use it on any simply grilled chicken, fish, or meat.

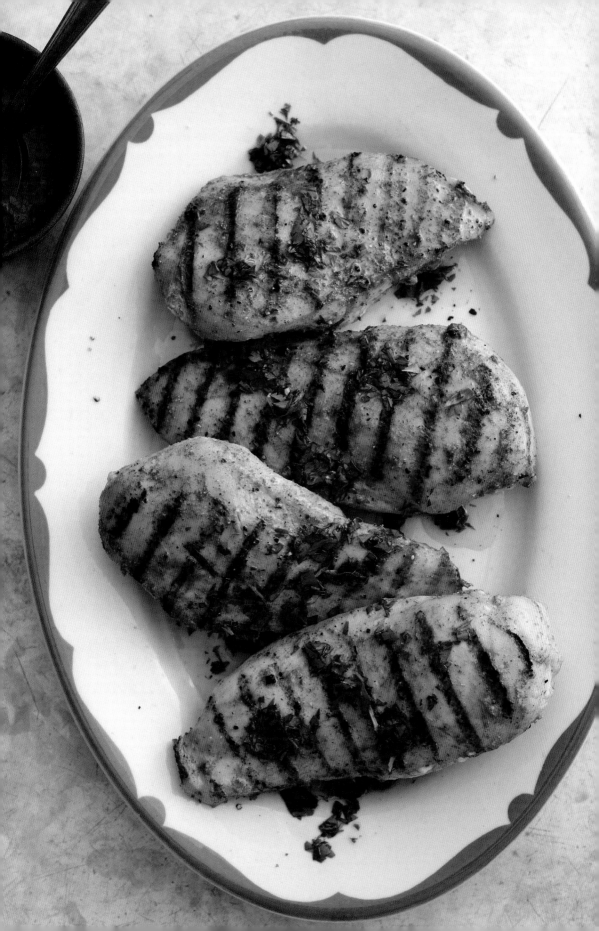

Tandoori-Style Baked Chicken

Hands-On Time: 10 minutes | **Total Time:** 35 minutes plus marinating time and standing time | **Makes:** 4 servings

Any chance you get to add a bit of turmeric to your diet enhances your health! Curcumin, the active ingredient in turmeric, provides antioxidants along with anti-inflammatory, antiviral, antibacterial, and anticancer effects. Serve this simple baked chicken with steamed green beans tossed with salt, pepper, and a little coconut oil. On Phase 3, you could serve it with ½ cup quick-cooking brown basmati rice; season the rice with some of the same spices used in the yogurt marinade.

BELLY BUDDIES:
Ginger, lime, Greek yogurt, turmeric, chicken breast

- 1 inch fresh ginger, peeled and cut into chunks
- 2 tablespoons fresh lime juice
- ½ cup nonfat plain Greek yogurt
- ½ teaspoon ground coriander
- ½ teaspoon ground cumin
- ½ teaspoon salt
- ¼ teaspoon turmeric
- ⅛ teaspoon ground allspice
- 4 boneless, skinless chicken breast halves (6 ounces each)

1. In a mini food processor, combine the ginger and lime juice and coarsely chop. Add the yogurt, coriander, cumin, salt, turmeric, and allspice and blend. Transfer the mixture to a nonaluminum baking dish just big enough to hold the chicken in one layer, such as a 7 x 11-inch glass baking dish.

2. Make several slashes on both sides of the chicken. Place it in the baking dish and turn to coat thoroughly with the yogurt mixture, rubbing it into the slashes. Set the chicken aside to marinate for 30 minutes. Meanwhile preheat the oven to 350°F.

3. Bake the chicken for 25 minutes, or until cooked through but still juicy (it will be faintly pink in the center). Let stand for 10 minutes before serving.

Per serving: 214 calories • 39g protein • 4.5g fat (1g saturated) • 0g fiber • 2g carbohydrate • 499mg sodium • 45mg magnesium

If you have gluten issues: Choose a gluten-free brand of Greek yogurt.

Cooking for One: Make the yogurt mixture using ¼ inch ginger; 1½ teaspoons lime juice; 2 tablespoons Greek yogurt; ⅛ teaspoon each coriander, cumin, and salt; a generous pinch of turmeric; and a small pinch of allspice. Use it to coat 1 chicken breast half. The baking time remains the same.

Lemon Chicken Under a Brick

Hands-On Time: 20 minutes | **Total Time:** 45 minutes | **Makes:** 4 servings

If you've got a brick, cover it with foil and use it here to weight down the chicken as it cooks. This helps the spices and lemon flavor get right into the chicken. Lemons are rich in flavonoids believed to help detoxify our body. This citrus fruit also contains vitamin C, an immune system booster, and potassium, a mineral that helps nerves and muscles communicate. Contrary to popular belief, there is no evidence that the acidity in lemons contributes to acid reflux. Lemons tenderize the chicken, perhaps actually making it easier to digest.

¾ teaspoon coarse (kosher) salt

½ teaspoon ground coriander

¼ teaspoon black pepper

4 bone-in, skin-on chicken breast halves (10 ounces each)

¼ cup fresh flat-leaf parsley leaves

2 lemons, 1 thinly sliced and 1 cut into wedges

1 tablespoon extra-virgin olive oil

BELLY BUDDIES: Chicken breast, lemon, olive oil

1. Preheat the oven to 375°F.

2. In a small bowl, combine the salt, coriander, and pepper.

3. Run your fingers under the skin of the chicken and lift it up, but do not remove it. Rub the flesh with the spice mixture, and top with the parsley and lemon slices. Pull the skin down over the lemon.

4. In a large ovenproof skillet, heat the oil over medium heat. Place the chicken, skin side down, in the skillet and place a heavy weight on top (another ovenproof pan will work). Cook for 5 minutes, then transfer the skillet to the oven (with the weight on top) and bake for 10 to 12 minutes, or until the skin is richly browned.

5. Remove the weight, turn the chicken over, and bake, uncovered, for 10 minutes longer, or until the chicken is cooked through. Remove the skin before eating. Serve with lemon wedges.

Per serving: 256 calories • 41g protein • 8g fat (2g saturated) • 0.5g fiber • 2g carbohydrate • 461mg sodium • 42mg magnesium

Cooking for One: Make the whole batch of the salt-coriander-pepper rub. Rub a 10-ounce bone-in, skin-on chicken breast half under the skin with a scant ½ teaspoon rub. Top the rub with 1 tablespoon parsley leaves and 2 to 3 lemon slices. Pull the skin back down over the lemon. Sear the chicken in ¾ teaspoon oil in a small skillet as directed, then bake as directed. Cooking times will be the same. Remove the skin before eating.

Chicken with Pipian Sauce

Hands-On Time: 20 minutes | **Total Time:** 30 minutes | **Makes:** 4 servings

Pipian sauce, a Mexican green sauce made with pumpkin seeds and spices, is often served over roast chicken. But it also works well over steamed vegetables or roast pork.

BELLY BUDDIES:
Pumpkin seeds, sesame seeds, tomato, olive oil, chicken breast

2½ tablespoons hulled pumpkin seeds (pepitas)

2 teaspoons sesame seeds

½ cup cilantro leaves and stems, plus leaves for garnish

1 plum tomato, coarsely chopped

1 teaspoon ground cumin

½ teaspoon salt

⅛ teaspoon cayenne pepper

2 teaspoons extra-virgin olive oil

4 boneless, skinless chicken breast halves (6 ounces each)

¾ cup low-sodium chicken broth (look for brands with no onions or garlic)

1. In a food processor, combine the pumpkin seeds, sesame seeds, cilantro, tomato, cumin, salt, and cayenne. Puree until very well combined. (The mixture will be slightly grainy due to the pumpkin and sesame seeds.)

2. In a large nonstick skillet, heat the oil over medium heat. Add the chicken and cook for 3 minutes per side, or until golden brown. Add the broth and pumpkin seed mixture and bring to a boil. Reduce to a simmer, cover, and cook, turning the chicken once in the sauce, for 7 minutes, or until the chicken is cooked through.

3. Serve the chicken with the sauce spooned over. Garnish with the cilantro leaves.

Per serving: 260 calories • 39g protein • 10g fat (2g saturated) • 1g fiber • 2g carbohydrate • 505mg sodium • 82mg magnesium

If you have gluten issues: Choose a gluten-free brand of chicken broth.

Cooking for One: Make the whole batch of sauce and freeze what you don't need in ⅓-cup portions. To make a single serving of chicken, in a small nonstick skillet, cook 1 chicken breast in ½ teaspoon oil until lightly browned. Add 3 tablespoons water and ⅓ cup pumpkin seed sauce, and cook until the chicken is just cooked through.

Braised Chicken with Tomatoes and Olives

Hands-On Time: 20 minutes | **Total Time:** 35 minutes | **Makes:** 4 servings

Braising, which is cooking in a small amount of liquid, produces chicken that is moist and tender. Serve with a side of steamed kale or sautéed spinach.

2 teaspoons extra-virgin olive oil

4 boneless, skinless chicken breast halves (6 ounces each)

⅓ cup low-sodium chicken broth (look for brands with no onions or garlic) or Homemade Chicken Broth (page 111)

1 can (14.5 ounces) no-salt-added diced tomatoes (look for brands with no onions or garlic)

½ cup no-salt-added canned chickpeas, drained and rinsed

¼ cup green olives, pitted and coarsely chopped

¼ teaspoon dried oregano

¼ teaspoon salt

½ cup coarsely chopped fresh flat-leaf parsley

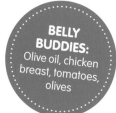

BELLY BUDDIES: Olive oil, chicken breast, tomatoes, olives

1. In a large nonstick skillet, heat the oil over medium heat. Add the chicken and cook for 3 minutes per side, or until lightly browned.

2. Add the broth to the skillet and bring to a simmer. Add the tomatoes, chickpeas, olives, oregano, and salt. Cover and simmer for 10 minutes, or until the chicken is cooked through. Transfer the chicken to a serving platter.

3. Increase the heat to high and bring the sauce in the pan to a boil. Boil for 5 minutes to concentrate the sauce. Stir in the parsley and spoon the sauce over the chicken.

Per serving: 280 calories • 39g protein • 7.5g fat (1.5g saturated) • 2.5g fiber • 11g carbohydrate • 435mg sodium • 59mg magnesium

If you have gluten issues: Choose a gluten-free brand of chicken broth.

Cooking for One: In a small skillet, heat ½ teaspoon oil and cook one 6-ounce boneless, skinless chicken breast half until browned. Add 1 chopped plum tomato, 2 tablespoons chickpeas, 1 tablespoon chopped olives, a pinch each of oregano and salt, and 2 tablespoons water. Simmer until the chicken is cooked through, then add 2 tablespoons chopped parsley.

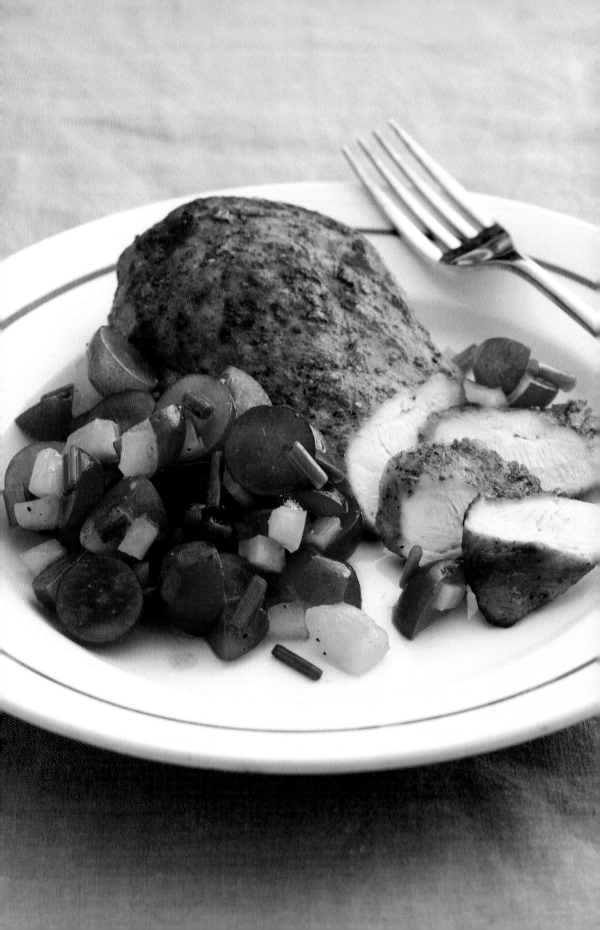

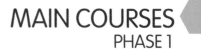

Spice-Rubbed Chicken with Grape Relish

Hands-On Time: 10 minutes | **Total Time:** 20 minutes | **Makes:** 4 servings

Garam masala, a mix of both sweet and savory Indian spices, gives you a jump start when making a rub. Red grapes provide resveratrol, a natural and powerful antioxidant that may reduce risk of cancer and inflammation. Serve the chicken with a simple tossed green salad and a small baked potato. If you're on Phase 3, serve with Cherry Tomato and Forbidden Rice Salad (page 230).

1½ teaspoons garam masala (look for brands with no onions or garlic)

½ teaspoon turmeric

¾ teaspoon coarse (kosher) salt

1 cup small seedless red grapes, quartered

½ cup finely diced yellow bell pepper

1 tablespoon snipped chives or sliced scallion greens

1 tablespoon red wine vinegar

2 teaspoons pure maple syrup

3 teaspoons extra-virgin olive oil

4 boneless, skinless chicken breast halves (6 ounces each)

BELLY BUDDIES: Turmeric, grapes, bell pepper, chives, maple syrup, olive oil, chicken breast

1. Preheat the broiler with the rack 4 inches from the heat.

2. In a small bowl, combine the garam masala, turmeric, and salt.

3. Measure out ¾ teaspoon of the spice mixture and transfer to a medium bowl. Add the grapes, bell pepper, chives, vinegar, maple syrup, and 1 teaspoon of the oil. Set the grape relish aside.

4. Rub the remaining spice mixture and the remaining 2 teaspoons oil onto both sides of the chicken. Broil, turning once, for 3½ minutes per side, or until the chicken is just cooked through but still juicy.

5. Top each chicken breast half with ⅓ cup grape relish.

Per serving: 266 calories • 37g protein • 8g fat (1.5g saturated) • 1g fiber • 10g carbohydrate • 560mg sodium • 51mg magnesium

If you have gluten issues: Choose a gluten-free brand of garam masala.

Cooking for One: Make the whole batch of spice rub and store it in a small jar in a cool place out of the sunlight. For a single serving of relish, combine ¼ teaspoon of the spice rub with ¼ cup grapes, 2 tablespoons diced yellow bell pepper, ¾ teaspoon each chives and red wine vinegar, ¼ teaspoon oil, and ½ teaspoon maple syrup. For the chicken, rub one 6-ounce boneless, skinless chicken breast half with ¼ teaspoon spice rub and ½ teaspoon oil. Broil as directed. Top with the grape relish.

Chicken Parmesan

Hands-On Time: 15 minutes | **Total Time:** 25 minutes | **Makes:** 4 servings

Chicken Parmesan is usually smothered under mozzarella and swimming in tomato sauce. Ours is a lighter, fresher version in which chicken is baked in a Parmesan crust and topped with broiled tomatoes. Serve with Tuscan Green Beans (page 238) and ½ cup cooked brown rice.

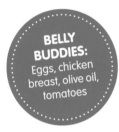

BELLY BUDDIES: Eggs, chicken breast, olive oil, tomatoes

½ cup brown rice flour

1 large egg white

2 teaspoons water

⅓ cup grated Parmesan cheese

¼ teaspoon salt

4 boneless, skinless chicken breast halves (6 ounces each)

Olive oil cooking spray

2 plum tomatoes, cut into 12 slices

1. Preheat the oven to 400°F.

2. Place ¼ cup of the rice flour in a shallow bowl or on a sheet of waxed paper. In a large shallow bowl, whisk together the egg white and water. In a third bowl, combine the cheese, salt, and remaining ¼ cup rice flour.

3. Dredge the chicken first in the plain flour, then in the egg mixture, and finally in the cheese mixture. Place the chicken on a baking sheet and coat generously with olive oil spray.

4. Bake for 10 minutes. Turn the oven to broil, top each chicken breast with 3 tomato slices, and broil 4 inches from the heat for 1 minute, or until the tomatoes are hot.

Per serving: 250 calories • 38g protein • 6g fat (2g saturated) • 0.5g fiber • 9g carbohydrate • 318mg sodium • 39mg magnesium

Cooking for One: Dredge one 6-ounce chicken breast half in 2 tablespoons rice flour, then in 1 large egg white beaten with 2 teaspoons water, and finally in a combination of 1 tablespoon rice flour, 1 rounded tablespoon cheese, and a pinch of salt. Bake as directed. Top with 3 slices plum tomato and broil for 1 minute.

Deviled Chicken

Hands-On Time: 10 minutes | **Total Time:** 35 minutes | **Makes:** 4 servings

Cayenne pepper makes this devilish, but feel free to go up or down according to your preference. Serve with Broccoli, Corn, and Grape Tomato Sauté (page 246).

2 (6-inch) corn tortillas

1 tablespoon plus 1 teaspoon olive oil mayonnaise (look for brands with no onions or garlic)

1 tablespoon plus 1 teaspoon Dijon mustard (look for brands with no onions or garlic)

½ teaspoon cayenne pepper

¼ teaspoon salt

4 boneless, skinless chicken breast halves (6 ounces each)

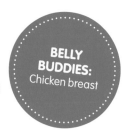

BELLY BUDDIES: Chicken breast

1. Preheat the oven to 400°F.

2. Place the tortillas on a baking sheet and bake for 10 minutes, or until crisp. (Leave the oven on.) Let the tortillas cool to room temperature, then break into pieces and process in a food processor until fine crumbs are formed.

3. In a small bowl, combine the mayonnaise, mustard, cayenne, and salt. Place the chicken breasts on a baking sheet and top each with the mayonnaise mixture, spreading it to coat the top. Scatter the tortilla crumbs over the mayo mixture, gently pressing to adhere.

4. Bake for 10 to 12 minutes, or until the top is lightly browned and the chicken is cooked through.

Per serving: 242 calories • 37g protein • 6g fat (1g saturated) • 0.5g fiber • 7g carbohydrate • 508mg sodium • 53mg magnesium

If you have gluten issues: Choose a gluten-free brand of mustard.

Cooking for One: Cut a 6-inch corn tortilla in half, and bake and process just one half as directed. Combine 1 teaspoon olive oil mayo, 1 teaspoon Dijon mustard, ⅛ teaspoon cayenne, and a pinch of salt and spread on one 6-ounce boneless, skinless chicken breast half. Bake as directed.

Roast Turkey Breast with Fresh Cranberry Relish

Hands-On Time: 25 minutes | **Total Time:** 1 hour 55 minutes | **Makes:** 8 servings

No need to wait until Thanksgiving—turkey breast is in the market all year long. Go for bone-in, skin-on turkey breast; the skin keeps the meat moist (remove it before you serve to avoid the fat), while the bone adds flavor. During the holiday season, pick up a few extra bags of cranberries and freeze them so you can prepare the relish any time. Cranberries, a rich source of proantho-cyanidins, lower your risk of gastric ulcers and urinary tract infections. Serve with Tuscan Green Beans (page 238) and a small baked potato.

BELLY BUDDIES: Orange, cranberries, grapes, maple syrup, turkey breast, olive oil

- ½ navel orange
- 2 cups fresh or frozen cranberries (8 ounces)
- ⅔ cup seedless red grapes, halved
- ⅓ cup pure maple syrup
- 1 3½-pound bone-in, skin-on turkey breast half
- 1 tablespoon poultry seasoning (look for brands with no onions or garlic)
- 1 teaspoon coarse (kosher) salt
- 1 tablespoon extra-virgin olive oil

1. Peel and coarsely chop the orange and place in a medium saucepan along with the cranberries, grapes, and maple syrup. Bring to a boil over medium heat, reduce to a simmer, and cook, stirring frequently, for 12 minutes, or until the cranberries have popped. Transfer to a bowl, cool to room temperature, and refrigerate until ready to use.

2. Preheat the oven to 400°F. Place the turkey in a small roasting pan. Run your fingers under the skin to separate it from the meat without removing it, and lift it up. Rub the flesh with the poultry seasoning, salt, and oil and replace the skin.

3. Roast for 15 minutes, or until the skin begins to color. Cover with foil and continue to roast, basting twice with the pan juices, for 1¼ hours, or until a thermometer registers 165°F.

4. To serve, remove the skin and carve the turkey into thick slices. Serve the relish alongside the turkey.

Per serving: 244 calories • 38g protein • 2.5g fat (0.5g saturated) • 1.5g fiber • 16g carbohydrate • 307mg sodium • 44mg magnesium

If you have gluten issues: Choose a gluten-free brand of poultry seasoning.

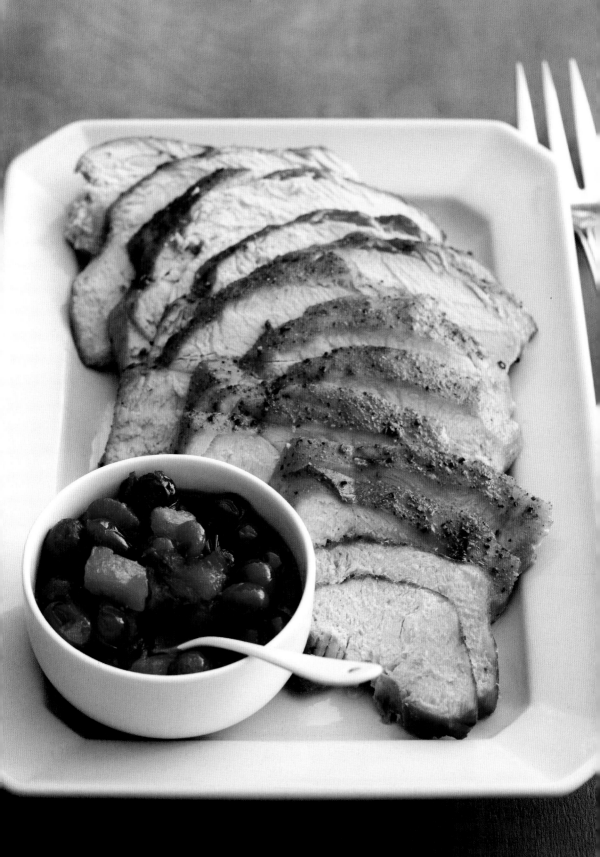

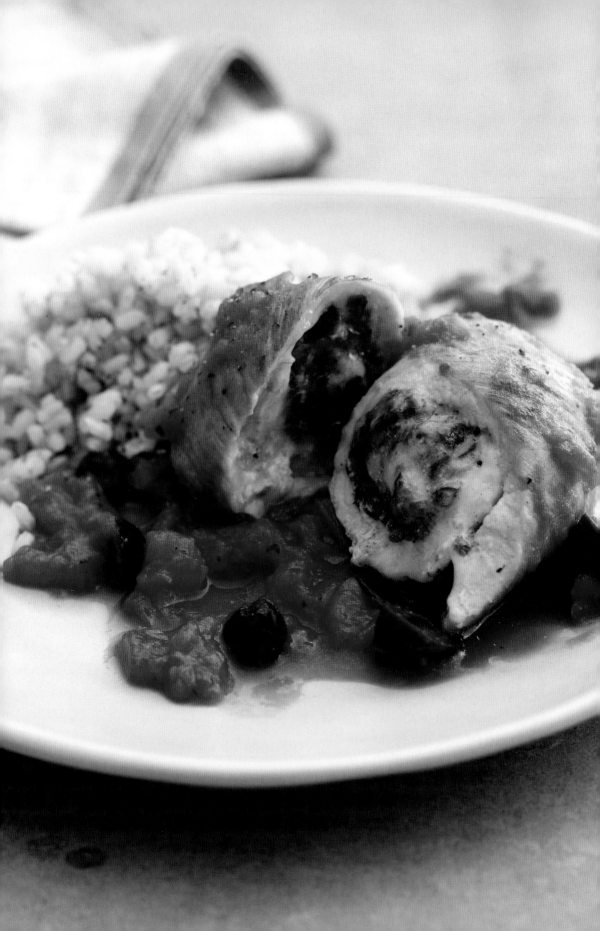

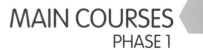

Turkey Braciole

Hands-On Time: 15 minutes | **Total Time:** 25 minutes | **Makes:** 4 servings

Braciole is an Italian dish of thin-sliced meat rolled around a stuffing. This version is braised in a tomato-y sauce and pairs well with ½ cup mashed potatoes (Phase 1), quinoa (Phase 2), or brown rice (Phase 3). For the half a package of spinach, use a serrated knife to saw the spinach in half while it's still frozen, then rewrap the portion you aren't using.

4 turkey breast steaks or cutlets (4 ounces each)

½ teaspoon ground sage

½ teaspoon coarse (kosher) salt

1 cup baby arugula

Half a 10-ounce package frozen chopped spinach, thawed and squeezed dry

½ cup reduced-fat Italian cheese blend

1 tablespoon extra-virgin olive oil

1 can (15 ounces) no-salt-added crushed tomatoes (look for brands with no onions or garlic)

¼ cup fresh orange juice

6 kalamata olives, pitted and coarsely chopped

BELLY BUDDIES: Turkey breast, arugula, spinach, olive oil, tomatoes, oranges, olives

1. Lay the turkey on a large cutting board. With a meat pounder or small heavy skillet, carefully pound the turkey to a rectangle about 6 x 4 inches. The turkey has a natural split on one side, so after pounding, overlap the meat at the split, which will keep the stuffing from falling out.

2. Sprinkle the cutlets on one side with the sage and salt. Cover with the arugula, then the spinach, and finally the cheese. Starting at a short end, carefully roll the turkey up (the ends will be open), taking care that it doesn't split open at the overlap. Secure the rolls with a toothpick or short wooden skewer.

3. In a large nonstick skillet, heat the oil over medium-high heat. Add the rolls and cook, without turning, for 2 minutes. Carefully flip the rolls and cook on the second side, without turning, for 2 minutes.

4. Reduce the heat to medium. Push the rolls to the sides of the pan and add the tomatoes, orange juice, and olives, stirring to combine. Move the rolls back into the center of the pan and spoon a little sauce on top. Bring to a simmer, cover, and cook for 10 minutes, or until the turkey is cooked through.

5. To serve, remove the toothpicks and spoon the sauce over the turkey rolls.

Per serving: 249 calories • 34g protein • 8g fat (2g saturated) • 2.5g fiber • 9g carbohydrate • 551mg sodium • 55mg magnesium

Turkey Cutlets in Spicy Peanut Sauce

Hands-On Time: 15 minutes | **Total Time:** 35 minutes | **Makes:** 4 servings

In Caribbean cooking, bananas are often used to thicken sauces and give them a natural sweetness. Here the banana rounds out the flavors of a peanut sauce, not to mention boosting its belly-friendly goodness. If you'd like, double the sauce to have extra to serve over brown rice.

BELLY BUDDIES: Tomatoes, banana, peanut butter, olive oil, turkey breast

- 1 cup canned no-salt-added diced tomatoes (look for brands with no onions or garlic)
- ⅓ cup water
- ½ medium banana, sliced
- ½ pickled jalapeño chile pepper, chopped
- 2 tablespoons creamy natural peanut butter
- 1 (6-inch) corn tortilla, torn into pieces
- 1 tablespoon white balsamic vinegar
- 1 teaspoon chili powder (look for brands with no onions or garlic)
- ½ teaspoon ground cumin
- ¾ teaspoon salt
- 1 tablespoon plus 1 teaspoon extra-virgin olive oil
- 4 turkey breast cutlets (4 ounces each)

1. In a small saucepan, combine the tomatoes, water, banana, chile pepper, peanut butter, tortilla, vinegar, chili powder, cumin, and salt. Bring to a boil and cook for 3 minutes to soften the tortilla. Transfer the mixture to a blender or food processor, and puree (or puree in the pan with an immersion blender).

2. Return the mixture to the saucepan, bring to a boil, reduce to a very low simmer, cover, and cook for 15 minutes to blend the flavors. Stir occasionally to make sure it's not sticking.

3. Meanwhile, in a large nonstick skillet, heat the oil over medium-high heat. Add the turkey and cook for 3 minutes, or until lightly browned on one side. Flip the turkey, add the sauce, and cook for 2 minutes, or until the turkey is cooked through.

Per serving: 261 calories • 31g protein • 9.5g fat (1g saturated) • 2g fiber • 13g carbohydrate • 573mg sodium • 10mg magnesium

If you have gluten issues: Choose a gluten-free brand of chili powder.

Cooking for One: Make the whole batch of sauce, portion out ½ cup, and cook a single turkey breast in 1 teaspoon oil in a small skillet. Freeze the remaining sauce in ½-cup portions.

Roast Salmon with Radish Raita

Hands-On Time: 15 minutes | **Total Time:** 25 minutes | **Makes:** 4 servings

In Indian cooking, raitas are cooling sauces meant to accompany spicy dishes. But this refreshing sauce also makes a lovely counterpoint to the richness of salmon. Salmon is one of the richest sources of heart- and tummy-friendly and inflammation-fighting omega-3 fats on earth!

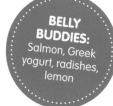

BELLY BUDDIES: Salmon, Greek yogurt, radishes, lemon

4 skin-on salmon fillets (5 ounces each)

¾ teaspoon coarse (kosher) salt

1 cup nonfat plain Greek yogurt

4 radishes, diced (½ cup)

3 tablespoons chopped fresh mint

1 tablespoon lemon juice

1. Preheat the oven to 450°F.

2. Place the salmon, skin side down, on a rimmed baking sheet and sprinkle the top with ½ teaspoon of the salt. Roast the salmon for 10 minutes, or until just cooked through but still moist.

3. Meanwhile, in a medium bowl, stir together the yogurt, radishes, mint, lemon juice, and the remaining ¼ teaspoon salt.

4. Lift the salmon off the skin (leaving it behind on the baking sheet) and place the fillets on 4 serving plates. Serve with the radish raita.

Per serving: 252 calories • 29g protein • 13g fat (2.5g saturated) • 0.5g fiber • 3g carbohydrate • 449mg sodium • 35mg magnesium

If you have gluten issues: Choose a gluten-free brand of Greek yogurt.

Cooking for One: Sprinkle one 5-ounce salmon fillet with ⅛ teaspoon coarse (kosher) salt. Combine ¼ cup nonfat plain Greek yogurt with 1 diced radish, 2½ teaspoons chopped fresh mint, and ¾ teaspoon lemon juice. Have the salmon with the radish raita.

Seared Mahi Mahi with Basil Oil

Hands-On Time: 15 minutes | **Total Time:** 25 minutes | **Makes:** 4 servings

Just a little bit of basil-infused olive oil goes a long way to make this fish extra tasty. It's also good drizzled on vegetables or tossed with a little gluten-free pasta. You can make a larger batch, strain it, and keep it in the refrigerator for up to 1 month. Serve the mahi mahi with Grilled Belgian Endives (page 234) and 4 small red potatoes per person.

BELLY BUDDIES: Olive oil, mahi mahi

⅓ cup packed fresh basil leaves

2½ tablespoons extra-virgin olive oil

4 skinless mahi mahi fillets (5 ounces each)

¾ teaspoon coarse (kosher) salt

½ teaspoon black pepper

1. In a small saucepan of boiling water, cook the basil leaves for 10 seconds to set their color. Drain and rinse under cold water. Squeeze dry and finely chop.

2. In a small skillet, heat the oil over low heat. Add the basil and cook for 3 to 4 minutes, or until the oil is fragrant. Set a fine-mesh sieve over a bowl and pour the oil through it, pressing on the basil to extract as much of the oil as possible.

3. Sprinkle the mahi mahi with the salt and pepper. Brush a grill pan with 1 teaspoon of the basil oil and heat over medium heat. Cook the mahi mahi for 5 minutes per side, or until just cooked through (timing will vary depending upon the thickness of the fish).

4. Place the fish on 4 serving plates and drizzle each serving with about 1½ teaspoons basil oil.

Per serving: 197 calories • 26g protein • 9.5g fat (1.5g saturated) • 0g fiber • 0g carbohydrate • 485mg sodium • 45mg magnesium

Cooking for One: Make the whole batch of oil. For a single serving of fish, heat ¼ teaspoon of the basil oil in a grill pan or small skillet, and cook one 5-ounce mahi mahi fillet. To serve, drizzle 1½ teaspoons basil oil over the fish.

Jerk Shrimp

Hands-On Time: 25 minutes | **Total Time:** 25 minutes | **Makes:** 4 servings

The jerk spice mixture, common in Jamaica, is a combo of hot and sweet spices. Cooking the shrimp over low heat keeps them from toughening up and getting chewy. Serve the shrimp with Kiwi and Orange Salad (page 220) or, if you're on Phase 3, Brown Rice Pilaf with Melted Carrots (page 257).

¾ teaspoon ground cumin

¾ teaspoon black pepper

½ teaspoon ground cinnamon

¼ teaspoon coarse (kosher) salt

¼ teaspoon ground allspice

⅛ teaspoon ground cloves

Pinch of cayenne pepper

1½ pounds large shrimp, peeled and deveined

4 teaspoons extra-virgin olive oil

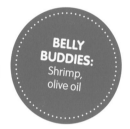

BELLY BUDDIES: Shrimp, olive oil

1. In a large bowl, combine the cumin, black pepper, cinnamon, salt, allspice, cloves, and cayenne. Add the shrimp and toss well to coat.

2. In a large nonstick skillet, heat 2 teaspoons of the oil over low heat. Add half the shrimp and cook for 2½ minutes per side, or until lightly browned and cooked through. Repeat with the remaining 2 teaspoons oil and shrimp.

Per serving: 196 calories • 32g protein • 7g fat (0.5g saturated) • 0.5g fiber • 1g carbohydrate • 487mg sodium • 1mg magnesium

Cooking for One: In a small bowl, combine ¼ teaspoon each cumin and black pepper, ⅛ teaspoon cinnamon, and a pinch each of salt, allspice, cloves, and cayenne. Toss the mixture with 6 ounces shrimp. In a small nonstick skillet, heat 1 teaspoon oil and cook the shrimp as directed.

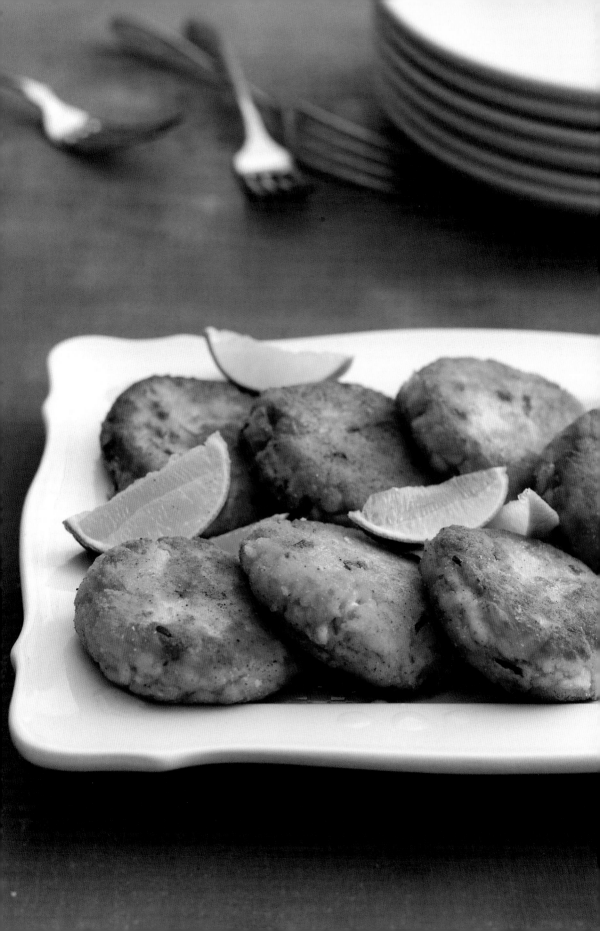

Crab Cakes

Hands-On Time: 15 minutes | **Total Time:** 35 minutes | **Makes:** 4 (2-cake) servings

Back fin crabmeat is less expensive than jumbo lump but still very tasty. The pieces are just smaller and may have more shell or cartilage in them. With either type of crab, make sure to pick through the pieces and discard any bits of shell. Serve with Home Fries (page 256) and Crisp Green Salad with Nuts in a Ginger Dressing (page 217).

¾ pound jumbo lump crabmeat or back fin

¼ cup light coconut milk

2 tablespoons snipped chives or sliced scallion greens

1 tablespoon fresh lime juice

1 tablespoon olive oil mayonnaise (look for brands with no onions or garlic)

2 teaspoons Dijon mustard (look for brands with no onions or garlic)

3 tablespoons extra-virgin olive oil

2 tablespoons coconut flour

Lime wedges

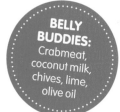

BELLY BUDDIES: Crabmeat, coconut milk, chives, lime, olive oil

1. In a large bowl, combine the crab, coconut milk, chives, lime juice, mayonnaise, and mustard. With your hands or a ¼-cup ice cream scoop, pack the mixture firmly into 8 patties.

2. In a large nonstick skillet, heat 1½ tablespoons of the oil over medium heat. Dredge 4 of the crab cakes in the coconut flour and cook for 3 to 5 minutes per side, or until golden brown and heated through (crabmeat is already cooked, so you're really just cooking the cakes until hot). Repeat with the remaining 1½ tablespoons oil and 4 crab cakes.

3. Serve with lime wedges for squeezing.

Per serving: 100 calories • 8g protein • 6.5g fat (1.5g saturated) • 0.5g fiber • 2g carbohydrate • 407mg sodium • 21mg magnesium

If you have gluten issues: Choose a gluten-free brand of mustard.

Cooking for One: Form all of the crab cakes and freeze those you aren't planning to eat right away (without coating them in coconut flour). When you are ready to cook the leftover crab cakes, there's no need to thaw. Just dredge in coconut flour and proceed with the recipe.

Cod Veracruz

Hands-On Time: 25 minutes | **Total Time:** 30 minutes | **Makes:** 4 servings

Cod fillets are one of the leanest and mildest flavored fish available in the sea. Here it's paired with canned fire-roasted tomatoes and jalapeño pepper to give this Mexican dish a deep tomato flavor and a spicy kick. That said, jalapeño peppers can be tricky—some are hot, others mild, so give the pepper a little taste before adding it to the sauce. Serve with Herbed Tricolor Quinoa (page 258).

BELLY BUDDIES: Olive oil, tomatoes, cod

5 teaspoons extra-virgin olive oil

1 jalapeño chile pepper, seeded and finely chopped (4 teaspoons)

1 can (14.5 ounces) no-salt-added diced fire-roasted tomatoes (look for brands with no onions or garlic)

½ teaspoon dried oregano

½ teaspoon salt

½ cup cilantro leaves and stems, coarsely chopped

3 tablespoons brown rice flour

4 skinless cod fillets (6 ounces each)

1. In a large nonstick skillet, heat 1 teaspoon of the oil over medium heat. Add the chile pepper and cook, stirring occasionally, for 2 minutes, or until tender. Add the tomatoes, oregano, and salt and bring to a simmer. Cook for 5 minutes, or until slightly reduced. Stir in the cilantro.

2. Place the rice flour in a shallow bowl. Dredge the cod in the flour, shaking off the excess. In a large nonstick skillet, heat 2 teaspoons of the oil over medium heat. Add 2 cod fillets and cook for 3 minutes per side, or until golden brown and cooked through. Repeat with the remaining 2 teaspoons oil and cod.

3. Serve the cod with the sauce spooned on top.

Per serving: 241 calories • 32g protein • 7g fat (1g saturated) • 1g fiber • 11g carbohydrate • 396mg sodium • 56mg magnesium

Cooking for One: In a small nonstick skillet, heat ¼ teaspoon oil over medium heat. Add 1 teaspoon chopped jalapeño, ½ cup chopped plum tomatoes, ⅛ teaspoon each oregano and salt, and 2 tablespoons chopped cilantro. Dredge 1 cod fillet in 2 teaspoons rice flour and cook in a medium nonstick skillet in 1 teaspoon oil. Spoon the sauce over the fish to serve.

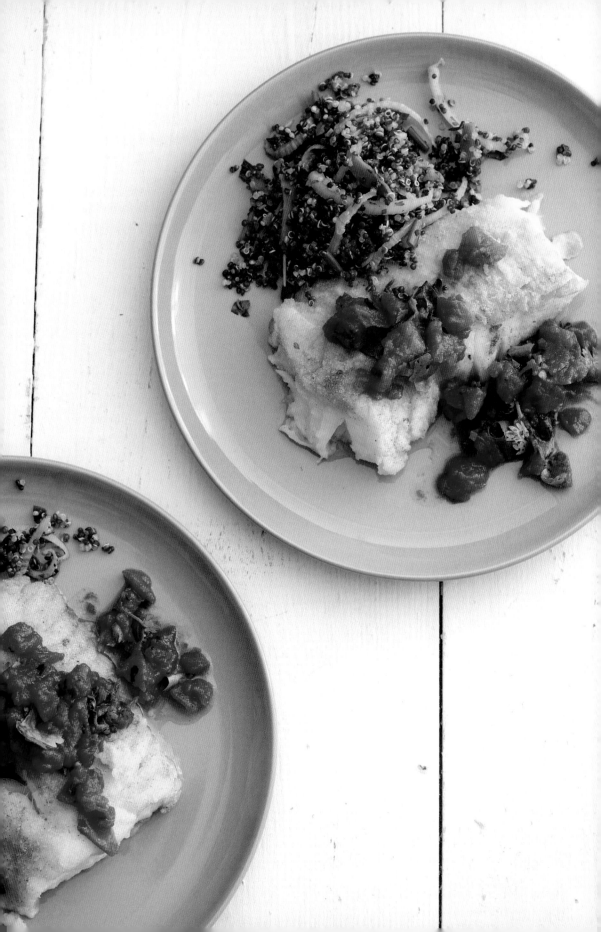

Potato and Cheese Frittata

Hands-On Time: 10 minutes | **Total Time:** 35 minutes | **Makes:** 4 (2-wedge) servings

A frittata, an Italian-style omelet, is equally good hot, at room temperature, or cold. So if you don't finish it for dinner, bring a wedge to work for lunch. Serve it (hot or cold) with Avocado, Tomato, Spinach, and Sprout Salad (page 218).

BELLY BUDDIES:
Potatoes, sweet potatoes, eggs, olive oil

¼ pound russet (baking) potatoes, peeled and sliced ¼ inch thick

¼ pound sweet potatoes, peeled and sliced ¼ inch thick

3 large eggs

2 large egg whites

½ teaspoon rubbed sage

¼ teaspoon salt

¼ teaspoon black pepper

½ cup shredded reduced-fat cheddar cheese

2 tablespoons grated Parmesan cheese

2 teaspoons extra-virgin olive oil

1. Preheat the oven to 350°F.

2. In a vegetable steamer, steam the russet and sweet potatoes for 5 minutes, or until tender.

3. In a large bowl, whisk together the whole eggs, egg whites, sage, salt, and pepper. Add the potatoes, cheddar, and Parmesan and stir to combine.

4. In a large nonstick ovenproof skillet, heat the oil over medium heat. Pour the mixture into the pan and cook, without stirring, for 3 minutes, or until the bottom has set.

5. Transfer to the oven and cook for 15 minutes, or until just set in the center. Cut into 8 wedges and serve.

Per wedge: 167 calories • 11g protein • 9g fat (3.5g saturated) • 1g fiber • 10g carbohydrate • 363mg sodium • 18mg magnesium

Cajun-Style Grilled Tofu Steaks with Pepper Relish

Hands-On Time: 20 minutes | **Total Time:** 20 minutes | **Makes:** 4 servings

Tofu takes on the flavors of the ingredients it is mixed with, so it makes a great base for the spicy pepper relish. Serve the tofu steak with a small baked sweet potato and Grilled Belgian Endives (page 234). You can make the tofu steaks up to 5 days ahead; store airtight, in a single layer, in the refrigerator. Serve them chilled or at room temperature.

- 2 containers (14 ounces each) extra-firm tofu
- 1 large red bell pepper, diced
- ¼ cup chopped fresh flat-leaf parsley
- 2 teaspoons chopped pickled jalapeño chile pepper
- ¾ teaspoon salt
- 1 teaspoon dried oregano
- 1 teaspoon dried thyme
- 1 teaspoon paprika
- ½ teaspoon cayenne pepper
- ¼ teaspoon black pepper
  Olive oil cooking spray

BELLY BUDDIES:
Tofu, bell pepper, olive oil

1. Halve each block of tofu horizontally into 2 slabs for a total of 4 "steaks." Set aside on paper towels to drain off a little moisture while you prep the remaining ingredients.

2. In a medium bowl, combine the bell pepper, parsley, chile pepper, and ¼ teaspoon of the salt and toss to coat.

3. In a small bowl, stir together the oregano, thyme, paprika, cayenne, black pepper, and the remaining ½ teaspoon salt. Rub the mixture onto both sides of the tofu steaks (about ½ teaspoon per side).

4. Heat a grill pan or cast-iron skillet over medium-high heat. Coat generously with cooking spray. Add the tofu steaks and cook for 4 minutes, or until browned on the first side. Flip the steaks and cook for 4 to 5 minutes, or until browned on the second side and heated through.

5. Slice the steaks on the diagonal and serve with the pepper relish.

Per serving: 216 calories • 21g protein • 11g fat (1.5g saturated) • 4g fiber • 8g carbohydrate • 464mg sodium • 8mg magnesium

If you have gluten issues: Choose a gluten-free brand of paprika.

Cooking for One: Make the full amount of relish. For the spice rub, divide all the ingredients in half. Use 1 block of tofu, cut in half as directed, and cook both steaks. Save the extra steak and relish for lunch.

Veggie Patties with Chipotle Mayo

Hands-On Time: 15 minutes | **Total Time:** 50 minutes | **Makes:** 4 servings

This recipe can be varied in many ways: Swap in pecans for the walnuts, kale or bok choy for the cabbage, or add some herbs such as basil, dill, or mint. Serve with a combo of sliced tomatoes and cucumbers. Tofu is great vegetarian protein for those with sensitive tummies, as the gas-producing GOS fibers in soybeans are minimized in processing.

BELLY BUDDIES: Tofu, oat bran, walnuts, bell pepper, cabbage, egg, olive oil

8 ounces extra-firm tofu, crumbled

½ cup oat bran

½ cup walnuts, finely chopped

1 red bell pepper, finely chopped

1 cup finely chopped cabbage (3 ounces)

1 large egg

½ teaspoon salt

1 tablespoon extra-virgin olive oil

2 tablespoons olive oil mayonnaise (look for brands with no onions or garlic)

¼ teaspoon chipotle chile powder

1. Preheat the oven to 350°F.

2. In a large bowl, combine the tofu, oat bran, walnuts, bell pepper, cabbage, egg, and salt until well combined. Pack the mixture into a ½-cup dry measuring cup, making 4 patties.

3. Place the patties on a baking sheet and drizzle the oil over them. Bake the patties, without turning, for 35 minutes, or until set.

4. Meanwhile, in a small bowl, stir together the mayonnaise and chile powder.

5. Serve the patties with a dollop of the chipotle mayonnaise.

Per serving: 242 calories • 12g protein • 18g fat (2.5g saturated) • 4.5g fiber • 14g carbohydrate • 383mg sodium • 36mg magnesium

If you have gluten issues: Choose a gluten-free brand of oat bran.

Cooking for One: Make all 4 patties and set aside one for cooking immediately. Refrigerate or freeze the remaining patties. Bake as directed in the recipe; the frozen patties, which can be baked from frozen, will need a few minutes longer in the oven. Either make the whole batch of chipotle mayo and store in the refrigerator, or make single portions as you go along: For each serving, mix 1½ teaspoons olive oil mayonnaise with a pinch of chipotle chile powder.

Red Quinoa Burger with Tzatziki

Hands-On Time: 20 minutes | **Total Time:** 40 minutes plus cooling time |
Makes: 4 servings

Tzatziki is a Greek yogurt dip/salad that is usually made with cucumber and garlic. We've omitted the garlic, subbed in zucchini instead of cucumber, and added dill for lots of flavor without FODMAPs. You can form the burger patties ahead of time. Refrigerate for up to 3 days or freeze for up to 1 month. Cook them when you want (no need to thaw the frozen ones). Serve with Moroccan Carrot Salad (page 229).

⅔ cup red quinoa

¾ cup nonfat plain Greek yogurt

1 teaspoon grated lemon zest

2 teaspoons fresh lemon juice

½ teaspoon dried oregano, crumbled

1 zucchini (5 ounces), grated on the large holes of a box grater and squeezed dry

¾ cup plus 2 tablespoons chopped fresh dill

1⅓ cups water

¼ teaspoon salt

½ cup crumbled reduced-fat goat cheese

1 large egg

1 large egg white

1 tablespoon extra-virgin olive oil

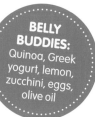

BELLY BUDDIES: Quinoa, Greek yogurt, lemon, zucchini, eggs, olive oil

1. Soak the quinoa in a bowl of cold water while you make the tzatziki.

2. In a small bowl, combine the yogurt, lemon zest, lemon juice, and oregano. Add the zucchini and 2 tablespoons of the dill. Refrigerate the tzatziki until ready to use.

3. In a medium saucepan, bring the water to a boil over medium heat. Drain the quinoa and add to the boiling water along with the salt. Reduce to a simmer, cover, and cook for 15 minutes, or until the quinoa is tender. Cool to room temperature.

4. Preheat the oven to 375°F.

5. Stir the goat cheese, whole egg, egg white, and remaining ¾ cup

dill into the quinoa. Pack tightly into a ½-cup measuring cup to make 4 mounds.

6. In a large nonstick skillet, heat the oil over medium heat. Add the mounds and flatten slightly with a spatula. Cook for 2 minutes, or until golden brown. Turn the patties over and cook for 2 minutes, or until golden brown.

7. Transfer to a baking sheet and bake for 5 minutes, or until cooked through. Serve with the tzatziki.

Per serving: 215 calories • 13g protein • 8g fat (1.5g saturated) • 2g fiber • 25g carbohydrate • 255mg sodium • 13mg magnesium

If you have gluten issues: Choose a gluten-free brand of Greek yogurt.

Japanese Dinner Pancake (Okonomiyaki)

Hands-On Time: 20 minutes | **Total Time:** 35 minutes | **Makes:** 4 servings

Okonomiyaki in Japanese means "as you like it," so feel free to switch around some of the ingredients to make this the way you'd like. You can go for more egg whites rather than whole eggs, or swap in bell pepper for the carrot. Just keep the green cabbage for its crunch and structure.

BELLY BUDDIES: Eggs, cabbage, carrot, ginger, chives, olive oil

⅓ cup brown rice flour

2 large eggs

4 large egg whites

⅓ cup water

1 tablespoon plus 1 teaspoon gluten-free reduced-sodium tamari

¼ teaspoon salt

2 cups shredded cabbage

1 carrot, shredded

1 cup no-salt-added canned chickpeas, mashed with a spoon or potato masher

3 tablespoons finely chopped fresh ginger

1½ tablespoons snipped chives or sliced scallion greens

1 tablespoon plus 1 teaspoon extra-virgin olive oil

1. Preheat the oven to 375°F.

2. In a large bowl, whisk together the rice flour, whole eggs, egg whites, water, tamari, and salt.

3. Stir in the cabbage, carrot, chickpeas, ginger, and chives.

4. In a large cast iron or nonstick ovenproof skillet, heat the oil over medium-low heat. Add the mixture and cook, without stirring, for 5 minutes, or until starting to set around the edges. Transfer the pan to the oven and cook for 12 to 15 minutes, or until set.

5. Run a metal spatula around the edge of the skillet and slide the pancake onto a platter, or cut into wedges and serve right from the skillet.

Per serving: 226 calories • 13g protein • 8g fat (1.5g saturated) • 4g fiber • 26g carbohydrate • 503mg sodium • 35mg magnesium

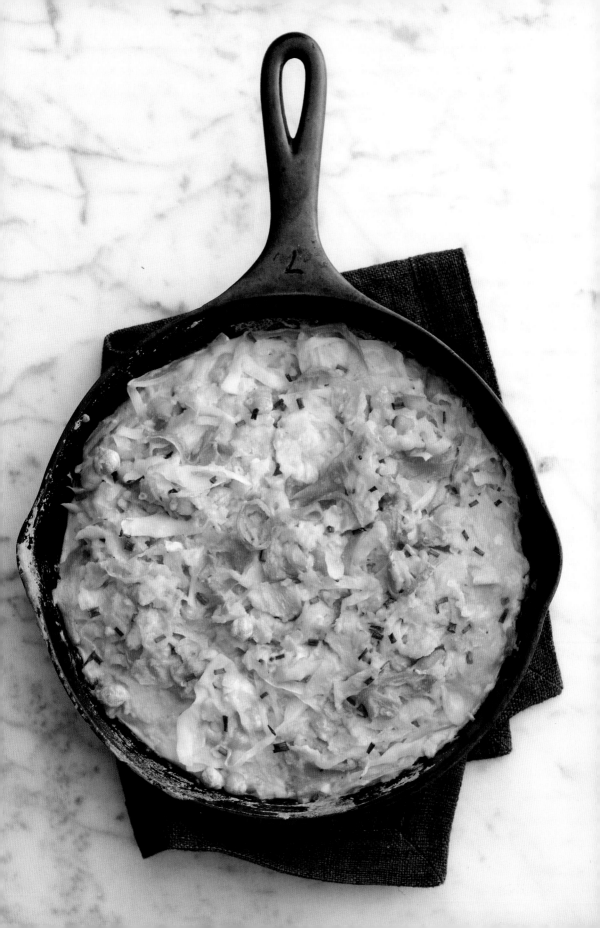

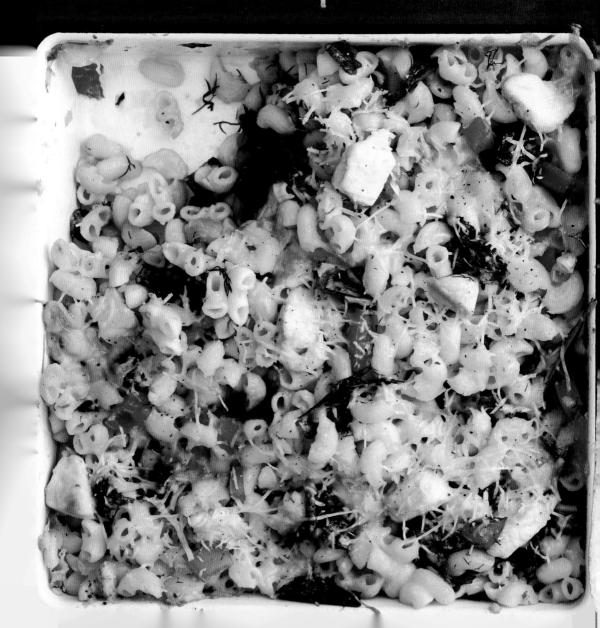

Sure to be a
crowd-pleaser!

Chapter 7

One-Dish Mains

All the belly-flattening goodness in one pot

Chicken Mac n' Cheese

Hearty Tomato-Basil Beef Stew

Hands-On Time: 20 minutes | **Total Time:** 25 minutes | **Makes:** 4 (2-cup) servings

This stew can be made a day ahead and reheated. This filling stew provides a hefty dose of vitamin C via the bell peppers, potatoes, and tomatoes. Vitamin C may protect against *H. pylori,* a gut bacterium linked with stomach ulcers and cancer.

BELLY BUDDIES: Potatoes, celery root, lean beef, olive oil, bell peppers, tomatoes

¾ pound red potatoes, cut into ⅓-inch dice

1 small celery root (¾ pound), peeled and cut into ⅓-inch dice

¼ cup cornmeal

¾ teaspoon salt

½ teaspoon black pepper

¾ pound well-trimmed beef sirloin, cut into ⅓-inch chunks

1 tablespoon plus 1 teaspoon extra-virgin olive oil

2 large orange bell peppers, diced

1 can (15 ounces) no-salt-added crushed tomatoes (look for brands with no onions or garlic)

2 cups low-sodium chicken broth (look for brands with no onions or garlic)

2 teaspoons grated orange zest (optional)

½ teaspoon dried oregano

½ cup minced fresh basil

1. In a large pot of boiling water, cook the potatoes and celery root for 5 minutes. Drain and set aside.

2. Meanwhile, in a shallow bowl, combine the cornmeal, ¼ teaspoon of the salt, and ¼ teaspoon of the pepper. Dredge the beef in the cornmeal mixture, shaking off the excess.

3. In a large nonstick saucepan or Dutch oven, heat 1 tablespoon of the oil over medium-high heat. Add the beef and cook, stirring frequently, for 1 to 2 minutes, or until browned all over. Transfer the beef to a plate.

4. Add the remaining 1 teaspoon oil to the pan. Add the bell peppers and ¼ teaspoon of the salt and cook, stirring frequently, for 4 minutes, or until crisp-tender.

5. Stir in the tomatoes, broth, orange zest (if using), oregano, and the remaining ¼ teaspoon salt and ¼ teaspoon pepper. Bring to a boil and cook for 2 minutes to meld the flavors. Add the beef, potatoes, celery root, and basil. Return to a simmer and cook for 3 minutes, or until the beef is just cooked through.

Per serving: 316 calories • 23g protein • 8g fat (2g saturated) • 6g fiber • 37g carbohydrate • 534mg sodium • 94mg magnesium

If you have gluten issues: Choose a gluten-free brand of chicken broth.

Sancocho Beef Stew

Hands-On Time: 20 minutes | **Total Time:** 20 minutes | **Makes:** 4 (1-cup) servings

Sancocho is a traditional Latin American soup/stew made of meat, vegetables, and often plantains. We've used a banana instead of the plantain as it's both easier to find and easier on your tummy. Plaintains are a significant source of highly fermentable, gas-producing resistant starch.

2 cups low-sodium beef broth (look for brands with no onions or garlic)

2 plum tomatoes, coarsely chopped

2 carrots, thinly sliced

1 tablespoon no-salt-added tomato paste (look for brands with no onions or garlic)

¾ teaspoon ancho chile powder

½ teaspoon salt

1 cup frozen corn kernels

1 tablespoon cornmeal mixed with 2 tablespoons water

¾ pound flank steak, thinly sliced across the grain, and cut into bite-size pieces

1 large banana, halved lengthwise and thickly sliced crosswise

1 cup cilantro leaves

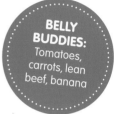
BELLY BUDDIES: Tomatoes, carrots, lean beef, banana

1. In a large skillet, bring the broth, tomatoes, carrots, tomato paste, chile powder, and salt to a boil over high heat.

2. Reduce to a simmer, add the corn, and cook for 1 minute. Add the cornmeal mixture and simmer for 2 minutes, or until lightly thickened. Add the meat and simmer for 1 minute, or just until cooked through.

3. Remove from the heat, divide among 4 serving bowls, and top with the banana slices and cilantro leaves.

Per serving: 223 calories • 22g protein • 5.5g fat (2g saturated) • 3.5g fiber • 23g carbohydrate • 444mg sodium • 52mg magnesium

If you have gluten issues: Choose a gluten-free brand of beef broth.

Cooking for One: In a medium skillet, heat ½ cup broth with ¼ cup chopped tomato, ½ sliced carrot, ¾ teaspoon tomato paste, ⅛ teaspoon each chile powder and salt. Add ¼ cup corn kernels, 3 ounces sliced flank steak, and ¾ teaspoon cornmeal mixed with 1½ teaspoons water. Top with ¼ sliced banana and ¼ cup cilantro leaves.

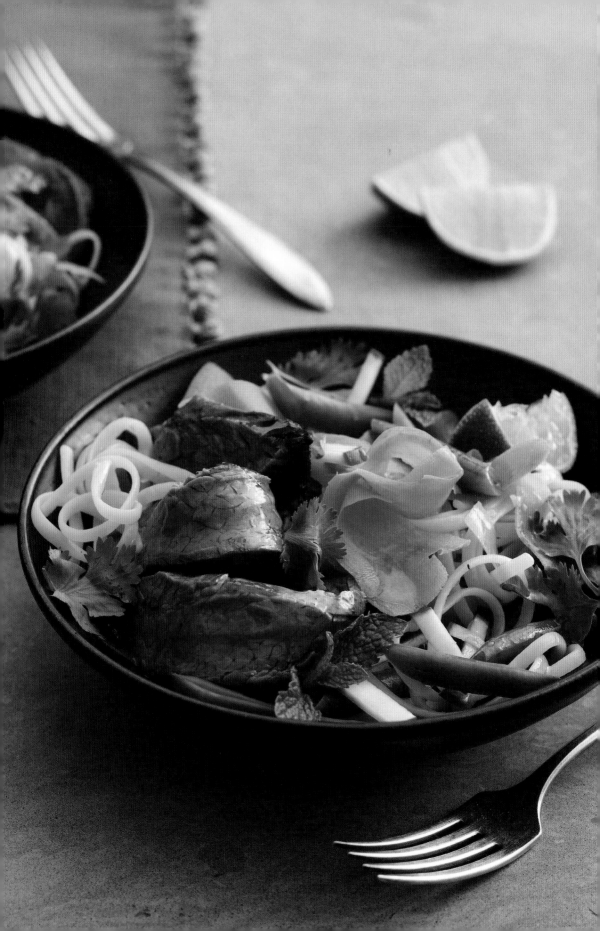

Thai Beef Salad

Hands-On Time: 25 minutes | **Total Time:** 35 minutes | **Makes:** 4 (1½-cup) servings

While cilantro and mint leaves are often chopped before being added to a dish, they've been left whole here—think of them the way you might salad greens. In the height of summer, when basil is in abundance, add some of those leaves, too.

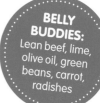

BELLY BUDDIES: Lean beef, lime, olive oil, green beans, carrot, radishes

- ¾ pound flank steak
- 3 tablespoons fresh lime juice
- 1 tablespoon plus 1 teaspoon extra-virgin olive oil
- ½ teaspoon coarse (kosher) salt
- ¼ teaspoon black pepper
- ½ pound green beans, cut into 1-inch lengths
- 2 ounces brown rice linguine

- 1 tablespoon reduced-sodium tamari or soy sauce
- 1 large carrot, shredded or shaved
- 3 radishes, cut into matchsticks (⅓ cup)
- ½ cup cilantro leaves
- ½ cup mint leaves
- Lime wedges

1. Preheat the broiler with the rack 4 inches from the heat. Place the flank steak on the broiler pan and rub it with 1 tablespoon of the lime juice, 1 teaspoon of the oil, ¼ teaspoon of the salt, and the pepper.

2. Broil for 7 minutes, without turning the steak, or until cooked to medium-rare (or more or less time depending on how you like your steak cooked). Cool to room temperature, then thinly slice across the grain.

3. Meanwhile, in a large pot of boiling water, cook the green beans until crisp-tender, 2 to 3 minutes (timing will vary depending on the thickness of the beans). Scoop them out with a slotted spoon and rinse under cold water to stop the cooking.

4. Add the linguine to the same pot of boiling water and cook according to package directions. Drain, rinse under cold water, and drain well.

5. In a large bowl, whisk together the tamari and the remaining 2 tablespoons lime juice, 1 tablespoon oil, and ¼ teaspoon salt. Add the steak, green beans, linguine, carrot, radishes, cilantro, and mint and toss well to combine. Serve with lime wedges.

Per serving: 251 calories • 22g protein • 10g fat (2.5g saturated) • 3.5g fiber • 19g carbohydrate • 487mg sodium • 45mg magnesium

If you have gluten issues: Choose a gluten-free brand of tamari.

Beef and Cabbage Stir-Fry with Sesame Quinoa

Hands-On Time: 15 minutes | **Total Time:** 25 minutes | **Makes:** 4 servings

The best way to cut flank steak for stir-fry is to first put it in the freezer for about 20 minutes to firm up (this makes it easier to slice). Cut the steak lengthwise (with the grain) into 2- to 3-inch-wide strips; then cut each strip across the grain into very thin slices. Ginger not only imparts flavor to this Asian-inspired dish, but also acts as a digestive aid, helping the stomach empty.

BELLY BUDDIES: Quinoa, ginger, lean beef, sesame seeds, olive oil, bell pepper, green cabbage

- ⅔ cup quinoa
- 1 tablespoon grated fresh ginger
- 2 tablespoons gluten-free reduced-sodium tamari
- 1 tablespoon dry sherry, white wine, or water
- ¼ teaspoon cayenne pepper
- ¾ pound flank steak, cut into thin slices for stir-fry

- 1⅓ cups water
- ¼ teaspoon salt
- 2 teaspoons sesame seeds, preferably black
- 1 tablespoon extra-virgin olive oil
- 1 yellow, orange, or red bell pepper, slivered
- 3 cups shredded green cabbage or coleslaw mix

1. In a medium bowl of water, soak the quinoa while you prepare the ingredients for the stir-fry.

2. In another medium bowl, combine the ginger, tamari, sherry, and cayenne. Add the beef to the bowl, tossing to coat.

3. Drain the quinoa and transfer to a saucepan. Add the 1⅓ cups water and salt. Bring to a boil, reduce to a simmer, cover, and cook for 15 minutes, or until tender. Stir in the sesame seeds and cover to keep warm.

4. Meanwhile, in a large nonstick skillet, heat the oil over medium-high heat. Add the beef and stir-fry for 1 to 2 minutes, or until lightly browned on the outside, but still pink. With a slotted spoon, transfer the beef to a plate.

5. Add the bell pepper and stir-fry until it starts to soften, about 1 minute. Add the cabbage and toss to combine. Cover and cook for 1 to 2 minutes, or until the cabbage and bell pepper are crisp-tender.

6. Return the beef to the skillet and cook just long enough to heat through. Serve over the quinoa.

Per serving: 302 calories • 25g protein • 11g fat (2.5g saturated) • 3g fiber • 26g carbohydrate • 561mg sodium • 32mg magnesium

Red Pork Chili with Parsnips and Chickpeas

Hands-On Time: 20 minutes | **Total Time:** 35 minutes | **Makes:** 4 (1¼-cup) servings

Pork tenderloin often comes in packages of two, so once opened, use what you need and freeze the remainder in 3- to 4-ounce serving portions. You can wrap the individual portions in butcher's wrap, or wrap in waxed paper or parchment and then overwrap in foil; remember to label and date. Frozen, the pork will keep up to 3 months. We included just enough chickpeas for belly-friendly fiber and just a little tomato paste for flavor—but not too much of either, which could bring on the bloat.

BELLY BUDDIES:
Olive oil, lean pork, parsnips

- 4 teaspoons Roasted Garlic Oil (page 54) or extra-virgin olive oil
- ½ pound parsnips, cut into ½-inch-thick slices
- 1¼ cups low-sodium chicken broth (look for brands with no onions or garlic) or Homemade Chicken Broth (page 111)

- ¾ pound pork tenderloin, cut into ½-inch chunks
- 3 tablespoons no-salt-added tomato paste (look for brands with no onions or garlic)
- 1 teaspoon ancho chile powder
- ¾ teaspoon coarse (kosher) salt
- 1 cup no-salt-added canned chickpeas, drained and rinsed

1. In a large skillet, heat 2 teaspoons of the oil over medium heat. Add half the pork and cook for 1 to 2 minutes, or until browned, turning the pieces as they color. Transfer the pork to a plate. Repeat with the remaining 2 teaspoons oil and pork. Return the first batch of pork to the pan.

2. Add the parsnips to the pan and cook for 2 minutes. Stir in the broth, tomato paste, chile powder, and salt and bring to a simmer. Cover and cook, stirring occasionally, for 10 to 12 minutes, or until the pork is tender.

3. Add the chickpeas and cook, stirring, for 2 minutes, or until heated through.

Per serving: 250 calories • 23g protein • 7g fat (1.5g saturated) • 5.5g fiber • 23g carbohydrate • 465mg sodium • 63mg magnesium

If you have gluten issues: Choose a gluten-free brand of chicken broth.

Cooking for One: In a small skillet, brown 3 ounces pork tenderloin in 1 teaspoon oil. Add 2 ounces parsnips, ⅓ cup broth, 2¼ teaspoons tomato paste, ¼ teaspoon each ancho powder and salt and simmer until tender. Add ¼ cup chickpeas and cook until heated through.

Roast Pork and Winter Vegetables

Hands-On Time: 20 minutes | **Total Time:** 1 hour | **Makes:** 4 servings

Acorn squash, white turnips, and potatoes make this a hearty, filling dish. Look for acorn squash in the fall or winter when it is at its most flavorful. If you don't have a mortar and pestle, the fennel seeds can be crushed by placing them in a resealable plastic bag and running a rolling pin back and forth across them. The roasted lemon bits give a little tang to the dish, but feel free to omit them if you prefer.

BELLY BUDDIES: Lean pork, olive oil, fennel, white turnips, potatoes

- ½ teaspoon fennel seeds, crushed
- ½ teaspoon crumbled dried rosemary
- 1 bay leaf, crumbled
- ½ teaspoon coarse (kosher) salt
- 1 pound pork tenderloin
- 1 tablespoon plus 1 teaspoon extra-virgin olive oil
- 1½ cups sliced fresh fennel

- 1 cup chunks (½ inch) skin-on acorn squash (about 5 ounces)
- ½ pound white turnips, peeled and cut into ½-inch chunks
- ½ pound small red or white potatoes, scrubbed and cut into 1-inch chunks
- 1 lemon, skin on, cut into ¼-inch dice and seeded

1. Preheat the oven to 375°F.

2. In a small bowl, combine the fennel seeds, rosemary, bay leaf, and ¼ teaspoon of the salt. Rub the mixture all over the pork along with 1 teaspoon of the oil. Set aside.

3. In a medium roasting pan, combine the fresh fennel, squash, turnips, potatoes, and lemon and drizzle with the remaining 1 tablespoon oil. Sprinkle the remaining ¼ teaspoon salt over the vegetables. Cover with foil and roast for 15 minutes.

4. Uncover, nestle the pork in the vegetable mixture, and roast, uncovered, for 25 minutes, or until the vegetables are tender and the pork registers 145°F when an instant-read thermometer is inserted into the thickest part of the meat.

Per serving: 245 calories • 26g protein • 7.5g fat (1.5g saturated) • 5g fiber • 20g carbohydrate • 367mg sodium • 63mg magnesium

Cooking for One: Make the entire dish and refrigerate the leftovers. Store the cooked pork unsliced until you're ready to carve off your portion for a lunch or even another dinner (it's great at room temp or chilled). Store the vegetables separately in 1-cup portions.

Southwestern Posole

Hands-On Time: 25 minutes | **Total Time:** 45 minutes | **Makes:** 4 (1¼-cup) servings

Canned hominy can usually be found alongside the canned vegetables or beans in the grocery store. If you've got some leftover hominy, pack it in an airtight freezer container and freeze it for another use; it'll keep for about 3 months. Use leftovers in place of corn in soups.

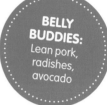

BELLY BUDDIES: Lean pork, radishes, avocado

1½ teaspoons chili powder (look for brands with no onions or garlic)

1 teaspoon ground cumin

2 cups low-sodium chicken broth (look for brands with no onions or garlic) or Homemade Chicken Broth (page 111)

½ teaspoon dried oregano

1½ cups canned hominy, drained and rinsed

¼ teaspoon salt

½ pound acorn squash, skin on, seeded, and cut into ½-inch chunks (1½ cups)

¾ pound boneless pork loin chops, cut into ½-inch-wide strips

4 radishes, thinly sliced (½ cup)

½ cup whole cilantro leaves

½ avocado, diced

Lime wedges

1. In a large skillet, toast the chili powder and cumin over low heat, stirring, for 1 minute, or until fragrant. Add the broth, oregano, and salt and bring to a boil.

2. Add the hominy and squash and reduce to a simmer. Cover and cook for 20 minutes, or until the squash is very tender.

3. Add the pork and simmer over very low heat, for 1 minute, or just until cooked through.

4. To serve, scatter the radishes, cilantro, and avocado over the top. Pass the lime wedges for squeezing.

Per serving: 290 calories • 28g protein • 12g fat (3.5g saturated) • 4g fiber • 17g carbohydrate • 456mg sodium • 58mg magnesium

If you have gluten issues: Choose gluten-free brands of chili powder and chicken broth.

Cooking for One: In a small skillet, toast ½ teaspoon chili powder and ¼ teaspoon ground cumin for 1 minute, or until fragrant. Add ½ cup chicken broth and ⅓ cup each hominy and acorn squash, cover, and simmer until tender. Add 3 ounces boneless pork loin and cook for 1 minute, or just until cooked through. Top with 1 sliced radish, 2 tablespoons cilantro leaves, ⅛ of an avocado, and a lime wedge.

Spinach, Pork, and Blueberry Salad

Hands-On Time: 15 minutes | **Total Time:** 40 minutes plus standing time |
Makes: 4 servings

Blueberries promote the growth of healthy gut bacteria that keep our tummies trim and happy. Mashing them here thickens the salad dressing while adding a slight sweetness. When shopping for Belgian endive, look for those that are white, with little or no yellowing at the tips.

BELLY BUDDIES:
Ginger, lean pork, olive oil, blueberries, spinach, Belgian endive

¾ teaspoon coarse (kosher) salt

¼ teaspoon ground ginger

¼ teaspoon ground allspice

¼ teaspoon black pepper

¾ pound pork tenderloin

5 teaspoons extra-virgin olive oil

1½ cups blueberries

2 teaspoons red wine vinegar

5 ounces baby spinach

1 Belgian endive, thickly sliced crosswise

2 ounces soft goat cheese, crumbled

1. Preheat the oven to 375°F.

2. In a large bowl, stir together the salt, ginger, allspice, and pepper. Measure out ¾ teaspoon of the mixture for the pork.

3. Place the pork in a small roasting pan and rub with the reserved spice mixture and 1 teaspoon of the oil.

4. Roast the pork for 25 minutes, or until it registers 145°F on an instant-read thermometer when inserted into the thickest part of the meat. Let stand for 10 minutes before cutting into ¼-inch-thick slices.

5. Add ½ cup of the blueberries to the large bowl with the spice mixture and mash with a potato masher or a fork. Stir in the vinegar and the remaining 4 teaspoons oil.

6. Add the spinach, endive, and remaining 1 cup blueberries to the dressing and toss to coat. Add the pork and any juices that have accumulated, and toss again.

7. Divide among 4 plates and scatter each serving with ½ ounce of goat cheese.

Per serving: 232 calories • 22g protein • 11g fat (3.5g saturated) • 4g fiber • 13g carbohydrate • 515mg sodium • 32mg magnesium

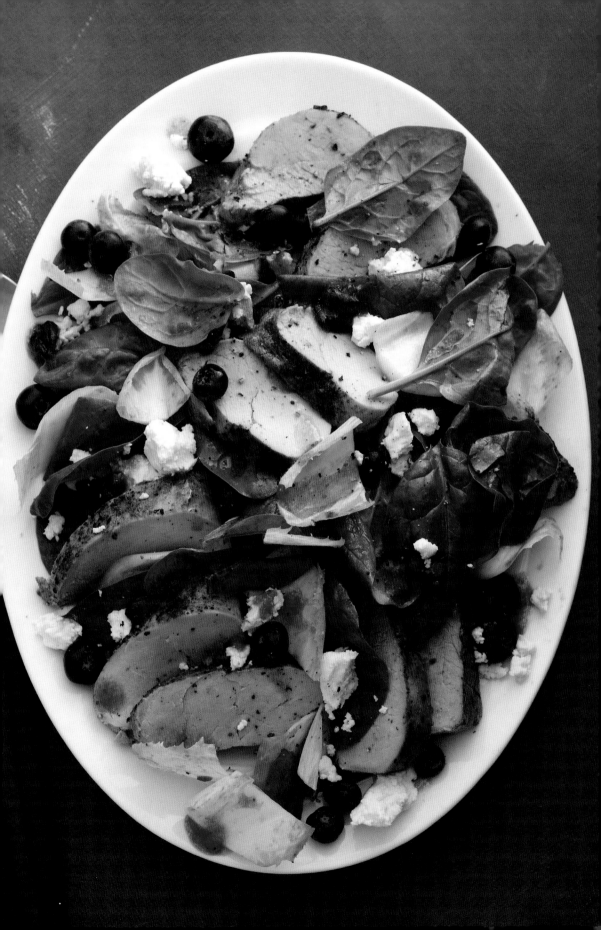

BBQ Pork Salad

Hands-On Time: 15 minutes | **Total Time:** 1 hour plus standing time | **Makes:** 4 servings

You can make the barbecue sauce well ahead and refrigerate. Bring back to room temperature before using. A splatter screen is a useful tool to have when you're cooking a thick sauce like this—you can keep it from spitting all over and at the same time allow steam to escape so you can reduce the sauce a bit. Contrary to popular belief, the common green cabbage used in this recipe is not a major gas producer. In fact, it's lower in FODMAPs compared to Napa or savoy cabbage, making it gentler on your tummy.

BELLY BUDDIES: Tomatoes, lean pork, olive oil, sweet potatoes, bell pepper, green cabbage

- 1 can (15 ounces) no-salt-added crushed tomatoes (look for brands with no onions or garlic)
- 2 tablespoons dark brown sugar
- ½ teaspoon salt
- ¼ teaspoon black pepper
- 3 tablespoons distilled apple cider vinegar
- 2 teaspoons mild chili powder (look for brands with no onions or garlic)
- 1½ teaspoons ground cumin
- 1 tablespoon extra-virgin olive oil
- 1 pound pork tenderloin
- 1 pound sweet potatoes, peeled and cut into ½-inch cubes
- 1 large red bell pepper, cut into matchsticks
- 1 cup frozen corn kernels, thawed
- 3 cups shredded cabbage (¼ medium or ½ small head)

1. Preheat the oven to 400°F. Line a baking sheet with foil (for easier cleanup).

2. In a small saucepan, combine the tomatoes, brown sugar, salt, black pepper, 1 tablespoon of the vinegar, 1 teaspoon of the chili powder, and ½ teaspoon of the cumin. Puree with an immersion blender (or blend everything in a mini food processor before putting in the saucepan). Bring to a simmer over medium-low heat,

then reduce heat to low, partially cover, and cook for 10 minutes to concentrate the flavors.

3. Measure out ⅓ cup of the mixture to use as a baste for the pork. Let the rest of the mixture cool slightly, then whisk in the oil and the remaining 2 tablespoons vinegar. This is the salad dressing.

4. Rub both sides of the pork with the remaining 1 teaspoon chili powder and 1 teaspoon cumin and roast for 10 minutes. Brush the pork with half of the basting mixture, then roast for another 10 minutes. Brush with the remaining basting mixture and roast for 10 to 15 minutes longer, or until it registers 145°F on an instant-read thermometer when inserted into the thickest part of the meat. Let stand for at least 10 minutes, then thinly slice crosswise.

5. Meanwhile, in a steamer, cook the sweet potatoes for 5 minutes, or until firm-tender. Transfer to a large salad bowl. Add the bell pepper, corn, cabbage, and salad dressing, tossing to combine. (Add any juices from the cutting board, too.)

6. Serve the sliced pork on a bed of the vegetables. Serve warm or at room temperature.

Per serving: 344 calories • 29g protein • 7g fat (1.5g saturated) • 7.5g fiber • 41g carbohydrate • 410mg sodium • 100mg magnesium

If you have gluten issues: Choose a gluten-free brand of chili powder.

Pork, Kasha, and Kiwi Salad

Hands-On Time: 10 minutes | **Total Time:** 45 minutes | **Makes:** 4 servings

Kasha, which is roasted buckwheat groats, comes in different granulations, from whole grain to fine. If you choose another granulation, check the package for cooking times. We chose whole granulation here for its look and texture. Vitamin C–rich kiwifruit also contain the enzyme actinidin, which helps your body digest protein. The salad can be made up to a day ahead, but add the kiwi shortly before serving so the actinidin doesn't have time to break down the pork and turn it mushy.

BELLY BUDDIES: Lean pork, lime, kasha, olive oil, kiwi fruit, tomatoes

¾ pound pork tenderloin

1 tablespoon fresh lime juice

1 tablespoon Worcestershire sauce

½ cup whole granulation kasha (roasted buckwheat groats)

3 tablespoons rice vinegar

1 tablespoon plus 1 teaspoon Roasted Garlic Oil (page 54) or extra-virgin olive oil

2 teaspoons Dijon mustard (look for brands with no onions or garlic)

½ teaspoon salt

2 kiwifruits, peeled, quartered lengthwise, and cut crosswise into ½-inch pieces

1 cup small grape tomatoes, quartered lengthwise

1. Preheat the oven to 375°F.

2. Place the pork tenderloin in a small roasting pan and sprinkle with lime juice. Brush with the Worcestershire sauce. Roast for 30 minutes, or until an instant-read thermometer registers 145°F when inserted into the thickest part of the meat.

3. Meanwhile, in a medium pot of boiling water, cook the kasha for 6 minutes, or until tender. Drain well, but don't rinse.

4. In a large bowl, whisk together the vinegar, oil, mustard, and salt.

Add the still-warm kasha, kiwi, and tomatoes and toss to combine.

5. Let the pork rest for 5 minutes before cutting into bite-size pieces. Add the pork to the bowl and toss to combine.

Per serving: 244 calories • 21g protein • 6.5g fat (1.5g saturated) • 3.5g fiber • 25g carbohydrate • 441mg sodium • 76mg magnesium

If you have gluten issues: Choose gluten-free brands of Worcestershire sauce and mustard.

Middle Eastern Chicken Skillet Dinner

Hands-On Time: 20 minutes **Total Time:** 35 minutes | **Makes:** 4 servings

Ginger, coriander, turmeric, and cinnamon are used to give Middle Eastern flavor to a simple chicken dinner. Turmeric and cinnamon also fight inflammation, while ginger promotes digestion. And the best part is that it's all made in a single skillet for easy cleanup!

- 1 tablespoon plus 1 teaspoon extra-virgin olive oil
- 4 boneless, skinless chicken breast halves (6 ounces each)
- 1 carrot, thinly sliced
- 1 parsnip, thinly sliced
- 1 red bell pepper, cut into 2 x ½-inch strips
- 1 yellow bell pepper, cut into 2 x ½-inch strips
- ¾ teaspoon ground ginger
- ¾ teaspoon ground coriander
- ½ teaspoon turmeric
- ½ teaspoon ground cinnamon
- ½ teaspoon salt
- ¼ teaspoon black pepper
- 1 cup low-sodium chicken broth (look for brands with no onions or garlic) or Homemade Chicken Broth (page 111)
- 1 cup juice-packed canned pineapple chunks, drained

BELLY BUDDIES: Olive oil, chicken breast, carrot, parsnip, bell peppers, pineapple

1. In a large nonstick skillet, heat the oil over medium heat. Add the chicken and cook for 2 minutes per side, or until lightly browned. Transfer the chicken to a plate (it'll cook more later).

2. Add the carrot, parsnip, and bell peppers to the skillet and cook, stirring occasionally, for 5 minutes, or until crisp-tender.

3. Add the ginger, coriander, turmeric, cinnamon, salt, and pepper, stirring to coat. Add the broth and bring to a simmer. Return the chicken to the pan, cover, and simmer for 7 minutes, or until the chicken is just cooked through. Stir in the pineapple and serve hot.

Per serving: 325 calories • 38g protein • 10g fat (2g saturated) • 3.5g fiber • 19g carbohydrate • 521mg sodium • 71mg magnesium

If you have gluten issues: Choose a gluten-free brand of chicken broth.

Cooking for One: In a medium nonstick skillet, heat 1 teaspoon oil. Cook 1 chicken breast half until browned and set aside. Add 2 tablespoons each sliced carrot and parsnip and ½ red or yellow bell pepper (cut into strips). Sprinkle with ¼ teaspoon each ground ginger and coriander; ⅛ teaspoon each turmeric, cinnamon, and salt; and a pinch of black pepper. Add ¼ cup broth or water and simmer. Add ¼ cup canned pineapple chunks at the end.

Chicken-Stuffed Peppers with Feta

Hands-On Time: 15 minutes | **Total Time:** 45 minutes | **Makes:** 4 servings

Ground chicken is a lean yet moist and tasty protein source in this savory dish. Substitute it in any of your favorite recipes that feature ground beef to save on both fat and calories. All you need to go with these cute stuffed peppers is a big tossed salad. Try Arugula Salad with Pine Nuts and Parmesan (page 214).

BELLY BUDDIES: Bell peppers, olive oil, chicken breast, almonds

4 large yellow bell peppers

3 teaspoons extra-virgin olive oil

¼ teaspoon salt

½ pound ground chicken breast

⅓ cup very finely chopped almonds

1 large egg

2 teaspoons reduced-sodium tamari or soy sauce

1 tablespoon no-salt-added tomato paste (look for brands with no onions or garlic)

¼ cup crumbled reduced-fat feta cheese

1. Preheat the oven to 375°F. Line a 9 x 13-inch baking pan with foil (for easy cleanup).

2. Lay the peppers on their sides. Slice off the top one-third of the peppers, just above the stem, to make little "boats" for stuffing. Finely dice enough of the sliced-off pieces to get 1 cup. (Save any remaining pieces of pepper for a snack.)

3. Cut out the seeds and as much of the ribs as you can to make room for the stuffing. Place the pepper boats cut side down in the pan and bake for 10 minutes to soften. Remove from the oven and flip the peppers cut side up. Leave the oven on.

4. Meanwhile, in a large nonstick skillet, heat 2 teaspoons of the oil over medium-high heat. Add the diced pepper and salt and cook for 2 minutes to soften. Add the remaining 1 teaspoon oil and the chicken to the pan and cook, breaking the chicken into crumbles with a spoon, for 1 minute, or until still a little pink. Off the heat, stir in the almonds and let cool slightly.

5. In a small bowl, beat the egg with the tamari. Beat in the tomato paste. Stir into the chicken mixture.

6. Divide the stuffing evenly among the peppers. Cover the pan with foil and return to the oven. Bake for 20 minutes, or until the peppers are tender and the stuffing is cooked through.

7. Uncover and sprinkle the peppers with the feta. Re-cover and let sit at room temperature for 5 minutes before serving.

Per serving: 239 calories • 20g protein • 12g fat (2.5g saturated) • 3g fiber • 15g carbohydrate • 469mg sodium • 65mg magnesium

If you have gluten issues: Choose gluten-free brands of tamari.

Cooking for One: Leftovers will hold up well for a couple of days, but if it is impractical to make all of the peppers, make the whole amount of stuffing but just cut up one pepper (you will have less chopped pepper in the stuffing). Stuff and bake it. Freeze the leftover stuffing in ½-cup portions. Use the stuffing to make more stuffed peppers later, or heat it up and have alongside an egg white omelet for a hearty breakfast.

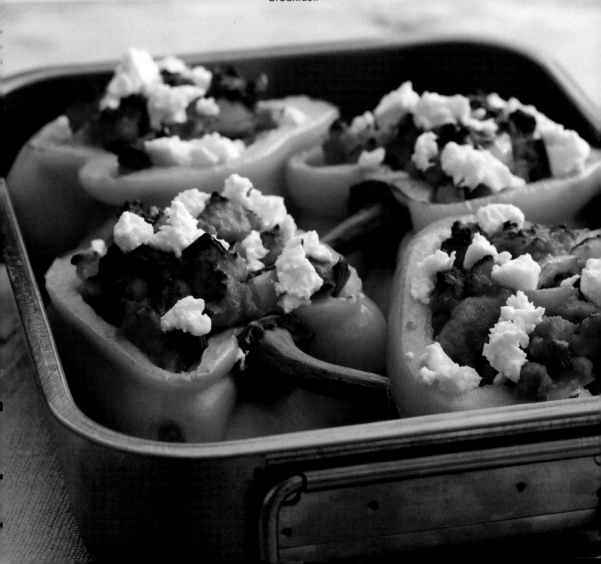

ONE-DISH MAINS
PHASE 3

Bibimbap

Hands-On Time: 15 minutes | **Total Time:** 30 minutes | **Makes:** 4 servings

Bibimbap is a popular Korean dish whose name means "mixed rice." The rice gets cooked, then vegetables are mixed in so they remain a little crunchy, and the whole thing is topped with fried eggs and chicken. The eggs provide a host of nutrients including stress-reducing B vitamins and inflammation-inhibiting vitamin D.

BELLY BUDDIES: Sesame oil, ginger, chicken breast, brown rice, spinach, carrots, bean sprouts, olive oil, eggs

- 3 tablespoons rice vinegar
- 1 tablespoon reduced-sodium tamari or soy sauce
- 1 tablespoon sesame oil
- ½ teaspoon ground ginger
- ¼ teaspoon black pepper
- ¾ pound boneless, skinless chicken breast

- 1⅓ cups water
- ⅔ cup quick-cooking brown rice
- 3 cups shredded fresh spinach
- 1 cup shredded carrots
- 1 cup bean sprouts
- 1 tablespoon extra-virgin olive oil
- 4 large eggs

1. In a large skillet, bring the vinegar, tamari, sesame oil, ginger, and pepper to a simmer over low heat. Add the chicken, cover, and simmer for 7 to 10 minutes, or until just cooked through. Reserving the pan juices, transfer the chicken to a cutting board and thinly slice crosswise.

2. Meanwhile, in a medium saucepan, bring the water to a boil. Add the rice and cook according to package directions. During the last minute of cooking, add the spinach, carrots, and bean sprouts to the rice. Stir in the reserved pan juices with a fork.

3. In a large nonstick skillet, heat the olive oil over medium heat. Add the eggs, cover, and cook for 3 minutes, or until the whites are set and the yolks are just set, but not hard.

4. Spoon the rice and vegetables onto a serving platter and top with the chicken and eggs.

Per serving: 308 calories • 28g protein • 14g fat (3g saturated) • 2.5g fiber • 17g carbohydrate • 530mg sodium • 55mg magnesium

If you have gluten issues: Choose gluten-free brands of tamari.

Cooking for One: In a small skillet, bring 2¼ teaspoons vinegar, ¾ teaspoon tamari, ¾ teaspoon sesame oil, ⅛ teaspoon ground ginger, and a pinch of pepper to a simmer. Add 3 ounces chicken breast and cook until done. Cook 3 tablespoons rice in ⅓ cup water until tender, adding ¾ cup shredded spinach, ¼ cup each carrots and bean sprouts, and the reserved chicken juices. Cook 1 egg in ¾ teaspoon olive oil and serve.

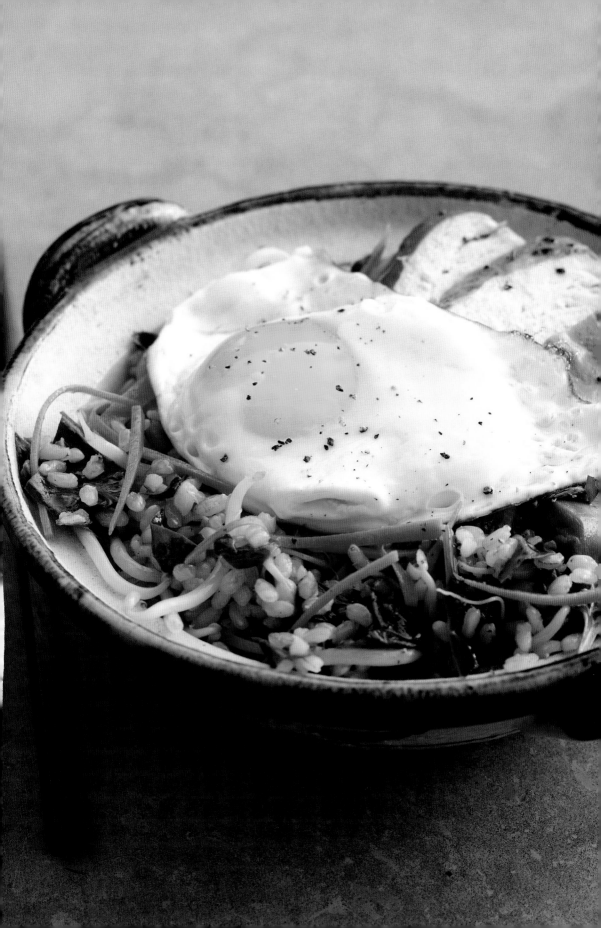

Arroz con Pollo

Hands-On Time: 15 minutes | **Total Time:** 30 minutes | **Makes:** 4 (1¾-cup) servings

Arroz con pollo (chicken and rice) is a classic dish that often has peas added to it. Here, we've used colorful kale instead, because it's lower in FODMAPs and provides added perks: It contains flavonol compounds kaempferol and quercetin, which may prevent growth of cancer cells and prevent inflammation.

BELLY BUDDIES:
Olive oil, brown rice, tomatoes, chicken breast, kale

1 tablespoon plus 1 teaspoon Roasted Garlic Oil (page 54) or extra-virgin olive oil

2 teaspoons smoked paprika

½ cup quick-cooking brown rice

1½ cups low-sodium chicken broth (look for brands with no onions or garlic) or Homemade Chicken Broth (page 111)

1 can (14.5 ounces) no-salt-added diced tomatoes (look for brands with no onions or garlic)

½ teaspoon salt

¼ teaspoon black pepper

1 pound boneless, skinless chicken breasts, cut into 1-inch chunks

4 cups shredded kale (½-inch-wide ribbons)

1. In a large saucepan, heat the oil over medium heat. Add the paprika and rice and stir to coat. Add the broth, tomatoes, salt, and pepper and bring to a boil. Reduce to a simmer, cover, and cook for 5 minutes.

2. Stir in the chicken and kale, cover, and cook for 10 minutes, or until the chicken is just cooked through and the dish is slightly saucy.

Per serving: 302 calories • 29g protein • 8.5g fat (1.5g saturated) • 3g fiber • 26g carbohydrate • 476mg sodium • 78mg magnesium

If you have gluten issues: Choose gluten-free brands of paprika and chicken broth.

Cooking for One: In a small saucepan, heat 1 teaspoon oil. Add ½ teaspoon smoked paprika and 2 tablespoons quick-cooking brown rice. Add 6 tablespoons broth, 1 chopped plum tomato, ⅛ teaspoon salt, and a pinch of pepper and cook for 3 to 5 minutes. Add ¼ pound chicken and 1 cup shredded kale and cook for 5 minutes, or until the chicken is cooked through.

North African Chicken Stew with Cilantro Couscous

Hands-On Time: 20 minutes | **Total Time:** 30 minutes | **Makes:** 4 (2¼-cup) servings

A variety of nutrient-dense low-FODMAP veggies and grains provide 7 grams of fiber in this filling and satisfying lightly spiced chicken dish.

⅔ cup brown rice couscous or quick-cooking brown rice

½ teaspoon salt

¼ cup chopped cilantro

1 tablespoon plus 1 teaspoon extra-virgin olive oil

4 large carrots, thinly sliced

1 large red bell pepper, diced

1 tablespoon chopped fresh ginger

3 cups low-sodium chicken broth (look for brands with no onions or garlic) or Homemade Chicken Broth (page 111)

2 yellow summer squash, quartered lengthwise and thinly sliced crosswise

1 cup dry white wine

2 teaspoons curry powder (look for brands with no onions or garlic)

¼ teaspoon cayenne pepper

1 pound boneless, skinless chicken breasts, cut into ½-inch chunks

¾ cup frozen green peas, thawed

Lime wedges

BELLY BUDDIES: Olive oil, carrots, bell pepper, ginger, summer squash, chicken breast

1. In a medium saucepan, cook the couscous according to package directions, using ¼ teaspoon of the salt. When it's done, stir in the cilantro and cover to keep warm.

2. Meanwhile, in a nonstick saucepan or Dutch oven, heat the oil over medium heat. Add the carrots, bell pepper, and ginger, stirring to coat. Add ½ cup of the broth, cover, and cook over low heat for 5 to 6 minutes, or until the carrots begin to soften.

3. Add the squash and the remaining ¼ teaspoon salt, re-cover, and cook for 2 minutes, or until the squash is crisp-tender.

4. Add the wine, curry powder, cayenne, and the remaining 2½ cups broth and bring to a simmer over medium-high heat. Stir in the chicken and peas and cook for 4 minutes, or just until the chicken is cooked through.

5. Serve the stew with a mound of couscous on the side, and lime wedges for squeezing.

Per serving: 399 calories • 31g protein • 9g fat (1.5g saturated) • 7g fiber • 40g carbohydrate • 539mg sodium • 64mg magnesium

If you have gluten issues: Choose gluten-free brands of chicken broth and curry powder.

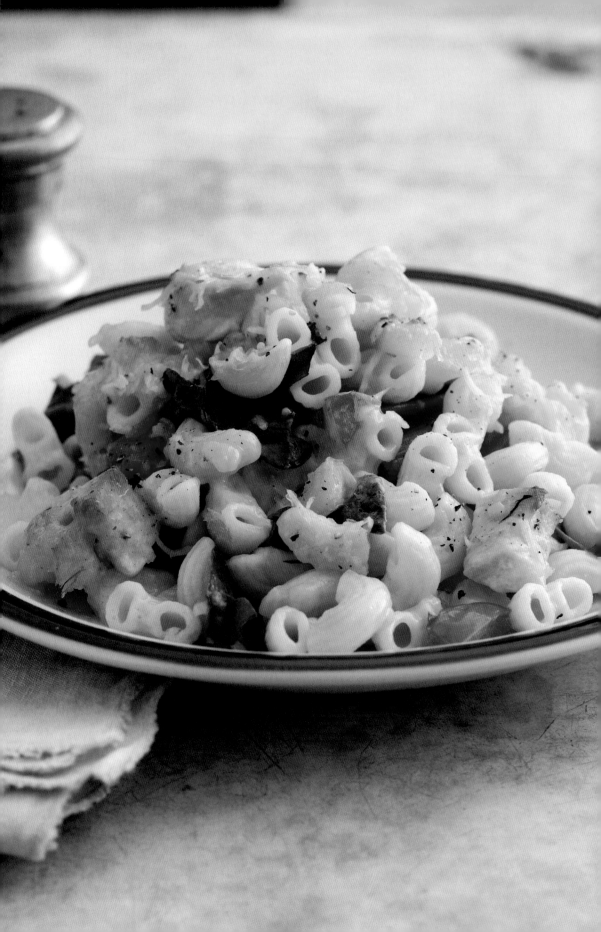

Chicken Mac and Cheese

Hands-On Time: 20 minutes | **Total Time:** 35 minutes | **Makes:** 4 servings

Cooking the pasta in broth gives extra flavor to this dish. By keeping the carb quantity small, we've reduced the carb density of this rich meal without losing any of its cheesy deliciousness. If you can find brown rice or quinoa-corn pasta, that lowers the carb density even more. Adding nourishing veggies and chicken boosts protein and fiber to keep you full longer.

2 cups low-sodium chicken broth (look for brands with no onions or garlic) or Homemade Chicken Broth (page 111)

1 cup water

4 ounces gluten-free macaroni

4 ounces Swiss chard, leaves and stalks thinly sliced (1 cup)

½ pound boneless, skinless chicken breast, cut into ½-inch chunks

2 cups shredded baby spinach (2 ounces)

2 plum tomatoes, coarsely chopped

¼ cup snipped fresh dill

¾ cup plus 2 tablespoons shredded reduced-fat cheddar cheese

¼ teaspoon black pepper

1 large egg

3 tablespoons grated Parmesan cheese

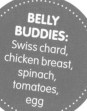

BELLY BUDDIES: Swiss chard, chicken breast, spinach, tomatoes, egg

1. Preheat the oven to 375°F.

2. In a medium saucepan, bring the broth and water to a boil over high heat. Add the macaroni and cook according to package directions, stirring occasionally, until a little shy of al dente. During the final 2 minutes of cooking, add the Swiss chard and chicken. Reserving the broth, drain the pasta mixture and transfer to a large bowl.

3. Add the spinach, tomatoes, dill, cheese, and pepper to the pasta.

Stir in the egg and ½ cup of the reserved broth.

4. Spoon the mixture into a 9 x 9-inch baking dish and sprinkle the Parmesan on top. Bake for 15 minutes, or until piping hot and the top is golden brown.

Per serving: 310 calories • 26g protein • 9.5g fat (5g saturated) • 2g fiber • 27g carbohydrate • 473mg sodium • 45mg magnesium

If you have gluten issues: Choose a gluten-free brand of chicken broth.

Chicken Enchiladas

Hands-On Time: 20 minutes | **Total Time:** 45 minutes plus standing time |
Makes: 4 servings.

You can cook and shred the chicken up to a day ahead and refrigerate it until you're ready to proceed with the recipe. If you like, add some cilantro leaves and finely diced red bell pepper to the tortillas before rolling them up.

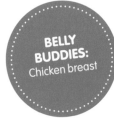

BELLY BUDDIES: Chicken breast

1½ cups low-sodium chicken broth (look for brands with no onions or garlic) or Homemade Chicken Broth (page 111)

1 teaspoon ground coriander

1 teaspoon ground cumin

½ teaspoon dried oregano

¼ teaspoon salt

1½ teaspoons ancho chile powder

¾ pound boneless, skinless chicken breasts, cut into large chunks

¼ cup no-salt-added tomato paste (look for brands with no onions or garlic)

4 (6-inch) corn tortillas

½ cup frozen corn kernels, thawed

¾ cup shredded reduced-fat cheddar cheese (3 ounces)

1. Preheat the oven to 350°F.

2. In a small saucepan, combine the broth, coriander, cumin, oregano, and salt and bring to a simmer over medium heat. Add the chicken, cover, and simmer for 5 to 10 minutes, or until the chicken is just cooked through and very faintly pink in the center.

3. Reserving the broth, transfer the chicken to a cutting board. When cool enough to handle, shred.

4. Whisk the tomato paste and chile powder into the reserved broth. Dip each tortilla into the broth mixture. Divide the

shredded chicken and corn among the 4 tortillas, roll them up, and place them, seam side down, in an 8 x 8-inch baking dish.

5. Pour the remaining broth mixture over the enchiladas and scatter the cheese over the top. Bake for 15 minutes, or until the cheese has melted and the tortillas are piping hot. Let rest in the pan for 10 minutes before serving.

Per serving: 274 calories • 28g protein • 8g fat (3.5g saturated) • 4g fiber • 23g carbohydrate • 468mg sodium • 57mg magnesium

If you have gluten issues: Choose a gluten-free brand of chicken broth.

Chicken Ambrosia

Hands-On Time: 25 minutes | **Total Time:** 30 minutes | **Makes:** 4 servings

Ambrosia salad (fruit, coconut, and marshmallows in a creamy dressing) was a fixture on dinner tables in the 1950s. Here the concept is adapted for a main-course salad—minus the marshmallows, of course. We've modernized the dressing, making it more tangy than sweet, and added pungent arugula to the salad. The Greek yogurt adds a nice dose of fat-free protein while minimizing tummy-troubling lactose.

BELLY BUDDIES: Olive oil, chicken breast, coconut, Greek yogurt, lemon, maple syrup, orange, pineapple, pecans, arugula

1 tablespoon plus 1 teaspoon extra-virgin olive oil

¾ pound boneless, skinless chicken breasts

3 tablespoons shredded unsweetened coconut

⅔ cup nonfat plain Greek yogurt

2 tablespoons fresh lemon juice

2 teaspoons pure maple syrup

½ teaspoon salt

¼ teaspoon black pepper

1 large navel orange, peeled and separated into segments (1 cup)

1 can (8 ounces) juice-packed pineapple chunks, drained

3 tablespoons coarsely chopped pecans

4 cups baby arugula

1. In a large nonstick skillet, heat 1 tablespoon of the oil over medium heat. Add the chicken and cook for 3½ minutes per side, or until golden brown and cooked through. When cool enough to handle, thinly slice crosswise.

2. In a small, dry skillet, toast the coconut over medium heat, tossing frequently, for 3 minutes, or until lightly browned.

3. In a large bowl, whisk together the yogurt, lemon juice, maple syrup, salt, pepper, and the remaining 1 teaspoon oil.

4. Add the orange segments, pineapple, pecans, and arugula and toss to combine.

5. To serve, divide the salad among 4 serving plates, top with the chicken, and sprinkle with the toasted coconut.

Per serving: 293 calories • 23g protein • 13g fat (4g saturated) • 3g fiber • 21g carbohydrate • 411mg sodium • 52mg magnesium

If you have gluten issues: Choose a gluten-free brand of Greek yogurt.

Grilled Chicken, Honeydew, and Avocado Salad

Hands-On Time: 25 minutes | **Total Time:** 25 minutes | **Makes:** 4 servings

Many supermarket produce departments sell cut-up honeydew, a source of anti-inflammatory magnesium. However, if you need to buy an entire melon to make this, cut up the extra and freeze it. You can then add the frozen chunks to a breakfast smoothie. Or you can puree the frozen melon with a squirt of lime juice in a food processor and serve it as a "sorbet."

BELLY BUDDIES: Olive oil, chicken breast, lemon, sesame oil, lettuce, honeydew melon, avocado

1 teaspoon curry powder (look for brands with no onions or garlic)

½ teaspoon salt

2 teaspoons plus 1 tablespoon extra-virgin olive oil

1¼ pounds boneless, skinless chicken breasts

2 tablespoons fresh lemon juice

2 teaspoons Dijon mustard (look for brands with no onions or garlic)

1 teaspoon sesame oil

6 cups shredded romaine lettuce

4 cups thinly sliced honeydew melon, cut to match the avocado slices (about 1 pound)

½ avocado, thinly sliced lengthwise and halved crosswise

1. Preheat the grill or a grill pan.

2. In a small bowl, stir together the curry powder and salt. Rub the chicken with 2 teaspoons of the olive oil. Rub the curry mixture into both sides of the chicken.

3. Grill the chicken for 5 to 6 minutes per side, or until cooked through but still juicy and a little pink in the center (the chicken will continue to cook as it rests). When cool enough to handle, thinly slice against the grain.

4. Meanwhile, in a small bowl, whisk together the lemon juice, mustard, sesame oil, and remaining 1 tablespoon olive oil.

5. Place the lettuce in a large bowl and toss with all but 2 tablespoons of the dressing.

6. To serve, make a bed of lettuce on each of 4 salad plates. Divide the chicken, melon, and avocado among the plates. Drizzle the remaining dressing over the salads.

Per serving: 286 calories • 32g protein • 14g fat (2g saturated) • 3g fiber • 10g carbohydrate • 532mg sodium • 59mg magnesium

If you have gluten issues: Choose gluten-free brands of curry powder and mustard.

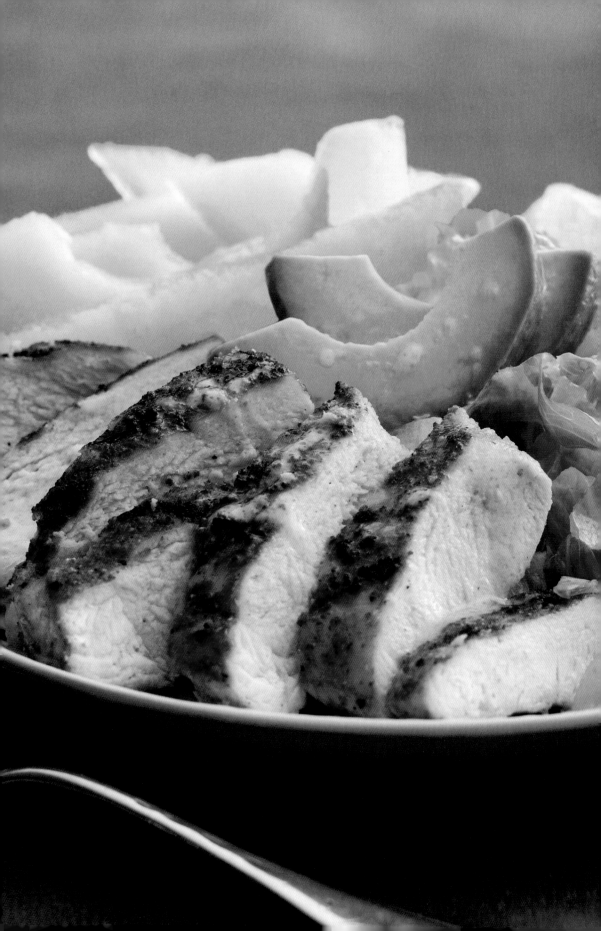

Asian Chicken Salad with Peanut Dressing

Hands-On Time: 25 minutes | **Total Time:** 30 minutes | **Makes:** 4 (2-cup) servings

You can use another salad green for the romaine lettuce, but try to find one that has a little crunch, like green cabbage. And if you can't find a Kirby cucumber, use a small regular cucumber; just be sure to seed it before slicing. If you have unsalted peanuts on hand, you can chop them and top each serving with a sprinkling (½ teaspoon) of them.

BELLY BUDDIES: Chicken breast, peanut butter, lime, sesame oil, bell pepper, cucumber, radishes, lettuce

1 cup low-sodium chicken broth (look for brands with no onions or garlic) or Homemade Chicken Broth (page 111)

½ cup water

¾ pound boneless, skinless chicken breasts

2 tablespoons natural creamy peanut butter

2 tablespoons fresh lime juice

2 teaspoons sesame oil

1 teaspoon ground coriander

½ teaspoon salt

1 red or orange bell pepper, cut into thin strips

1 Kirby cucumber, quartered lengthwise and thinly sliced

2 radishes, thinly sliced and cut into matchsticks (⅓ cup)

4 cups sliced romaine lettuce

1. In a medium saucepan, combine the broth and water and bring to a simmer over low heat. Add the chicken, cover, and simmer for 7 minutes, or until the chicken is just cooked through. Reserving the broth, transfer the chicken to a cutting board. When cool enough to handle, shred the chicken.

2. In a food processor, combine the peanut butter, lime juice, sesame oil, coriander, salt, and ¼ cup of the reserved broth and puree until smooth. Transfer to a large bowl.

3. Add the bell pepper, cucumber, radishes, and romaine to the bowl with the dressing. Add the chicken and toss to coat.

Per serving: 203 calories • 22g protein • 9g fat (1.5g saturated) • 3g fiber • 9g carbohydrate • 410mg sodium • 44mg magnesium

If you have gluten issues: Choose a gluten-free brand of chicken broth.

Cooking for One: Cook 3 ounces chicken in ½ cup broth. Reserve 2 tablespoons of the broth. Shred the chicken. Make the dressing: 1½ teaspoons peanut butter, 1½ teaspoons lime juice, ½ teaspoon sesame oil, ¼ teaspoon ground coriander, ⅛ teaspoon salt, and the reserved broth. Toss the dressing with ¼ cup pepper strips, ¼ cup cucumber slices, 1 small radish in matchsticks, 1 cup sliced romaine lettuce, and the shredded chicken.

Parmesan-Crusted Turkey Cutlets with Watercress Salad

Hands-On Time: 25 minutes | **Total Time:** 25 minutes | **Makes:** 4 servings

Crispy turkey cutlets are nestled under a bed of tangy watercress and tomatoes. The contrast—of cool on hot, and crisp on soft—is very nice indeed. Turkey breast cutlets are one of the leanest poultry protein sources, which means less calories and fat.

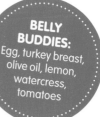

BELLY BUDDIES:
Egg, turkey breast, olive oil, lemon, watercress, tomatoes

1 large egg white

1 tablespoon water

⅔ cup grated Parmesan cheese

¼ cup plus 2 tablespoons potato starch

4 turkey breast cutlets or steaks (4 ounces each)

3 tablespoons extra-virgin olive oil

2 tablespoons fresh lemon juice

2 teaspoons Dijon mustard (look for brands with no onions or garlic)

¼ teaspoon salt

4 cups watercress (large stems removed), baby spinach, or baby arugula

3 plum tomatoes, cut into ½-inch chunks

1. In a shallow bowl, beat the egg white with the water. In a separate bowl, combine the cheese and ¼ cup of the potato starch. Place the remaining 2 tablespoons cornstarch in a third bowl. Dip the cutlets first in the plain potato starch, then in the egg white, then in the cheese mixture, patting it on to adhere.

2. In a large nonstick skillet, heat 1 tablespoon of the oil over medium-high heat. Add 2 cutlets and cook for 2 minutes per side, or until golden brown and crisp. Repeat with another 1 tablespoon of the oil and the remaining 2 cutlets.

3. In a large bowl, whisk together the lemon juice, mustard, salt, and the remaining 1 tablespoon oil until well combined. Add the watercress and tomatoes and toss to coat.

4. Serve each cutlet topped with a generous ½ cup salad.

Per serving: 334 calories • 35g protein • 15g fat (3.5g saturated) • 1g fiber • 15g carbohydrate • 542mg sodium • 19mg magnesium

If you have gluten issues: Choose a gluten-free brand of mustard.

Turkey Goulash with Broken Fettuccine

Hands-On Time: 25 minutes | **Total Time:** 40 minutes | **Makes:** 4 servings

Roasting your own peppers means you can completely control how much sodium you're getting. The peppers in a jar or from a supermarket olive bar are often packed in a light brine. You'll need 8 ounces of roasted pepper, which is about a cup.

BELLY BUDDIES: Bell peppers, Greek yogurt, olive oil, zucchini, turkey breast

- 2 large red bell peppers
- 1 tablespoon balsamic vinegar
- 1 tablespoon sweet paprika
- 1 tablespoon brown rice flour
- ½ cup nonfat plain Greek yogurt
- 8 ounces brown rice fettuccine, broken into thirds
- 2 tablespoons chopped fresh dill, plus extra for garnish

- 3 teaspoons extra-virgin olive oil
- ½ teaspoon salt
- 3 zucchini, cut into ½-inch cubes
- 1 cup low-sodium chicken broth (look for brands with no onions or garlic)
- ¾ pound turkey breast, cut into ½-inch chunks

1. Preheat the broiler.

2. Sit the peppers upright on a cutting board and cut them vertically into flat panels (discard the core and seeds). Arrange the pepper pieces on a broiler pan skin side up. Broil for 12 minutes, or until charred all over. Remove from the oven and flip the pepper pieces, skin side down, on the broiler pan to cool. When cooled, pull off and discard the skins.

3. In a blender or food processor, combine the roasted peppers, vinegar, and paprika and puree until smooth.

4. In a small bowl, stir the flour into ¼ cup of the yogurt.

5. In a large pot of boiling water, cook the pasta according to package directions. Drain, return to the pot, and toss with 1 tablespoon of the dill, 1 teaspoon of the oil, and ¼ teaspoon of the salt.

6. Meanwhile, in a nonstick saucepan or Dutch oven, heat the remaining 2 teaspoons oil over medium heat. Add the zucchini and the remaining ¼ teaspoon salt. Cover and cook for 2 minutes, stirring once or twice. Add the roasted pepper puree, broth, and remaining 1 tablespoon dill and bring to a simmer. Add the turkey and return to a simmer. Stir in the yogurt-flour mixture and cook, uncovered, for 3 minutes to thicken the sauce.

7. To serve, spoon the goulash over the noodles and serve with a dollop of the remaining ¼ cup yogurt. Garnish with the fresh dill.

Per serving: 401 calories • 31g protein • 5g fat (0.5g saturated) • 4g fiber • 54g carbohydrate • 406mg sodium • 28mg magnesium

If you have gluten issues: Choose gluten-free brands of paprika, Greek yogurt, and chicken broth.

Cooking for One: Make the whole goulash, and refrigerate or freeze the leftovers in 1¼-cup portions. For a single serving, cook 2 ounces brown rice fettuccine, drain, and toss with ¼ teaspoon oil, a pinch of salt, and 1 teaspoon chopped fresh dill.

Turkey and Shrimp Jambalaya

Hands-On Time: 35 minutes | **Total Time:** 50 minutes | **Makes:** 4 (1¾-cup) servings

A jambalaya is New Orleans' answer to a Spanish paella. This one is made with brown rice and turkey for a bit of a health makeover. Brown rice is 100 percent whole grain. Plus, it's high in belly-flattening magnesium!

BELLY BUDDIES: Brown rice, bell peppers, tomatoes, turkey breast, shrimp.

- 2¼ cups plus 2 tablespoons water
- 1 cup long-grain brown rice
- 1 teaspoon dried thyme
- ½ cup sliced scallion greens or chives
- 1 tablespoon plus 1 teaspoon extra-virgin olive oil
- ½ plus ⅛ teaspoon salt
  Black pepper

- 1 small fennel bulb, stalks discarded, cored and diced
- 2 large bell peppers (1 yellow, 1 orange), chopped
- 1 pint grape tomatoes, ½ finely chopped, ½ quartered
- ¾ pound turkey breast, cut into cubes
- ¼ pound peeled and deveined medium shrimp (40/50 count)

1. In a medium saucepan, combine 2¼ cups of the water, the rice, thyme, half of the scallions greens, 1 teaspoon of the oil, ½ teaspoon of the salt, and a generous amount of black pepper. Bring to a boil over high heat, then reduce to a simmer, partially cover, and cook for 25 minutes.

2. Meanwhile, in a nonstick soup pot or Dutch oven, heat the remaining 1 tablespoon oil over medium-high heat. Add the fennel and cook, stirring occasionally, for 3 to 4 minutes, or until it begins to brown. Add the bell peppers and 2 tablespoons water, reduce the heat to medium, cover, and cook for 5 minutes, or until the vegetables begin to soften.

3. Add the chopped tomatoes and the remaining ⅛ teaspoon salt and cook, uncovered, for 3 minutes, or until the tomatoes collapse.

4. Add the turkey and the rice (and any remaining cooking liquid) to the pot and stir well. Let the mixture come to a low simmer, then cover tightly and cook for 12 minutes, stirring once or twice.

5. Stir in the shrimp and quartered tomatoes. Cover and cook for 2 minutes, or until the shrimp are opaque. Serve the jambalaya sprinkled with the remaining scallion greens.

Per serving: 396 calories • 33g protein • 7g fat (1g saturated) • 7g fiber • 50g carbohydrate • 541mg sodium • 90mg magnesium

Creamy Fish Stew

Hands-On Time: 25 minutes | **Total Time:** 45 minutes | **Makes:** 4 (1½-cup) servings

We've used a skillet, instead of a saucepan, for this stew so the fish pieces would sit on top in a single layer and cook evenly. While some stews are thickened with the addition of eggs and oil, mayonnaise does the same trick. This is a delicious way to incorporate more heart-healthy fish into your diet.

1 tablespoon plus 1 teaspoon extra-virgin olive oil

½ pound small red or white potatoes, well scrubbed, cut into ½-inch chunks

1 cup diced fennel (4 ounces)

1 cup peeled and diced celery root (6 ounces)

½ cup thinly sliced carrot

½ teaspoon salt

3 cups water

1 teaspoon grated orange zest

1 pound skinless cod or grouper fillets, cut into large chunks

2 tablespoons olive oil mayonnaise (look for brands with no onions or garlic)

BELLY BUDDIES: Olive oil, potatoes, celery root, carrot, cod

1. In a large skillet, heat the oil over medium heat. Add the potatoes, fennel, celery root, and carrot and cook, stirring occasionally, for 5 minutes, or until the potatoes start to brown. Add the salt and 1 cup of the water, cover, and simmer for 5 minutes.

2. Add the orange zest and the remaining 2 cups water and bring to a boil. Reduce to a simmer, place the fish on top, cover, and cook for 7 minutes, or until the fish is opaque throughout. Whisk in the mayonnaise.

3. Serve in shallow soup bowls.

Per serving: 226 calories • 22g protein • 7.5g fat (1g saturated) • 3g fiber • 17g carbohydrate • 495mg sodium • 64mg magnesium

Cooking for One: In a small skillet, heat 1 teaspoon oil over medium heat. Add 2 small red potatoes, cut up, ¼ cup each diced fennel and celery root, and 2 tablespoons sliced carrot and cook for 5 minutes. Add ⅛ teaspoon salt and ¼ cup water, cover and simmer until tender. Add ¼ teaspoon grated orange zest, and ½ cup water. Place ¼ pound cod on top, cover and simmer until the fish is cooked through, about 5 minutes. Whisk in 1½ teaspoons olive oil mayonnaise.

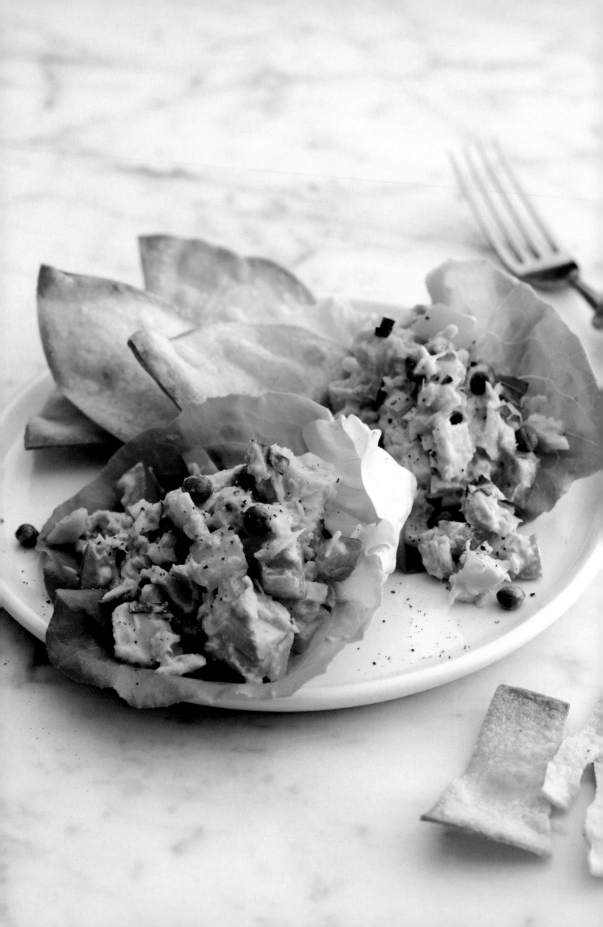

Tricked-Out Tuna Salad

Hands-On Time: 10 minutes | **Total Time:** 20 minutes | **Makes:** 4 (¾-cup) servings

This makes a fine salad for Phases 1 and 2, as long as you leave out the corn tortillas.

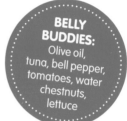

BELLY BUDDIES: Olive oil, tuna, bell pepper, tomatoes, water chestnuts, lettuce

- 4 (6-inch) corn tortillas
  Lemon juice, lime juice, or vinegar (any type), for brushing
  Olive oil cooking spray
- 2 pinches of salt
- 1 can (12 ounces) water-packed albacore tuna, drained and flaked
- ⅓ cup olive oil mayonnaise (look for brands with no onions or garlic)
- ¼ teaspoon black pepper

- 1 tablespoon coarsely chopped fresh tarragon leaves
- 1 small yellow bell pepper, diced
- 1 plum tomato, seeded and chopped
- ½ cup diced water chestnuts (2 ounces)
- 2 tablespoon capers, rinsed and drained
- 8 small Boston lettuce leaves

1. Preheat the oven to 350°F.

2. Lightly brush one side of the tortillas with the lemon or lime juice or vinegar, and coat lightly with the cooking spray. Sprinkle with the salt. Cut the tortillas into quarters, spread on a baking sheet, and bake for 7 to 10 minutes, or until crisp and golden.

3. In a large bowl, combine the tuna, mayonnaise, black pepper, and tarragon and mix well. Add the bell pepper, tomato, water chestnuts, and capers and toss gently to combine.

4. Scoop the tuna salad into lettuce cups and garnish with the tortilla quarters.

Per serving: 246 calories • 23g protein • 9g fat (1.5g saturated) • 3g fiber • 18g carbohydrate • 413mg sodium • 59mg magnesium

Cooking for One: Make the entire salad and save leftovers for lunch, but leave the tomato out of the salad—only add freshly chopped tomato as you eat the leftovers (it tends to get mushy as it sits). For the tortillas, you can make just one, or you can make the whole batch. Store them at room temperature, but re-crisp them in a toaster oven before serving.

Greek-Style Tuna Noodle Casserole

Hands-On Time: 25 minutes | **Total Time:** 45 minutes | **Makes:** 4 servings

Spinach, feta, oregano, and fresh dill give this take on a tuna noodle casserole a decidedly Greek feel. Canned tuna is a convenient way to up your omega-3 intake. Omega fats are well known for reducing inflammation.

BELLY BUDDIES:
Olive oil, bell pepper, spinach, tuna

4 ounces brown rice elbow macaroni

2 teaspoons extra-virgin olive oil

1 red bell pepper, cut into ½-inch squares

2 tablespoons brown rice flour

2 cups lactose-free 1% milk

½ teaspoon black pepper

¼ teaspoon dried oregano

1 package (10 ounces) frozen chopped spinach, thawed and squeezed dry

4 ounces reduced-fat feta cheese, crumbled

1 can (5 ounces) water-packed albacore tuna, drained

½ cup snipped fresh dill

1. Preheat the oven to 350°F.

2. In a pot of boiling water, cook the pasta according to package directions. Drain.

3. Meanwhile, in a large saucepan, heat the oil over medium heat. Add the bell pepper and cook, stirring occasionally, for 7 minutes, or until tender. Sprinkle with the flour, stirring to coat. Gradually whisk in the milk until smooth. Whisk in the black pepper and oregano and bring to a simmer. Cook, stirring occasionally, until the sauce is lightly thickened.

4. Add the spinach, feta, tuna, dill, and pasta to the sauce and stir until combined.

5. Spoon into a 9 x 9-inch baking dish and bake for 20 minutes, or until piping hot.

Per serving: 330 calories • 24g protein • 9g fat (4g saturated) • 4g fiber • 37g carbohydrate • 527mg sodium • 87mg magnesium

Fish Taco Salad

Hands-On Time: 30 minutes | **Total Time:** 40 minutes | **Makes:** 4 servings

While many fish tacos have cabbage and radishes, we've swapped in radicchio for both the crunch and the peppery taste. Yellow and red grape tomatoes make for a more colorful salad, but it will be just as good for your tummy if you use all yellow or all red tomatoes. In fact, any type of tomato works here.

2 (6-inch) corn tortillas

6 teaspoons fresh lime juice

5 teaspoons extra-virgin olive oil

1½ pounds skinless grouper fillet

½ teaspoon coarse (kosher) salt

1 teaspoon pure maple syrup

½ teaspoon chili powder (look for brands with no onions or garlic)

1 cup yellow grape tomatoes, halved

1 cup red grape tomatoes, halved

1½ cups shredded radicchio

½ cup sliced scallion greens or snipped chives

½ cup packed cilantro leaves

1 cup diced avocado

BELLY BUDDIES: Olive oil, grouper, maple syrup, tomatoes, avocado

1. Preheat the oven to 350°F.

2. Place the tortillas on a baking sheet and brush with 2 teaspoons of the lime juice and 1 teaspoon of the oil. Bake for 10 to 12 minutes, or until crisp. When cool enough to handle, break into pieces.

3. In a large nonstick skillet, heat 2 teaspoons of the oil over medium-low heat. Sprinkle the grouper with the salt and cook for 3 minutes per side, or until opaque throughout (timing will vary depending on the thickness of the fish). When cool enough to handle, break into bite-size pieces.

4. In a large bowl, whisk together the maple syrup, chili powder, and the remaining 4 teaspoons lime juice and 2 teaspoons oil. Add the grape tomatoes, radicchio, scallion greens, cilantro, and avocado and toss to combine.

5. Divide among 4 plates and top with the fish and tortilla chips.

Per serving: 331 calories • 36g protein • 13g fat (2g saturated) • 4.5g fiber • 17g carbohydrate • 345mg sodium • 79mg magnesium

If you have gluten issues: Choose a gluten-free brand of chili powder.

Margarita Shrimp Salad

Hands-On Time: 30 minutes | **Total Time:** 30 minutes | **Makes:** 4 servings

We've left out the tequila but have incorporated some of the other margarita ingredients—such as orange juice, lime juice, and, in the case of spicy margaritas, chipotle chile powder (smoky and hot). So, if you don't fancy spicy dishes, simply omit the chipotle powder.

BELLY BUDDIES: Orange, lime, shrimp, avocado, Greek yogurt, olive oil, Belgian endives, kiwifrui

¼ cup fresh orange juice

3 tablespoons fresh lime juice

½ teaspoon coarse (kosher) salt

1 pound large shrimp, peeled and deveined

⅓ cup diced avocado

⅓ cup nonfat plain Greek yogurt

2 tablespoons water

1 teaspoon chipotle chile powder

1 teaspoon no-salt-added tomato paste (look for brands with no onions or garlic)

4 teaspoons extra-virgin olive oil

3 Belgian endives (4 ounces each), halved lengthwise and thickly sliced crosswise

2 kiwifruit, peeled and diced

1. In a medium bowl, whisk together the orange juice, 1 tablespoon of the lime juice, and ¼ teaspoon of the salt. Add the shrimp and toss to coat.

2. In a food processor, combine the avocado, yogurt, water, chile powder, tomato paste, 2 teaspoons of the oil, and the remaining 2 tablespoons lime juice and ¼ teaspoon salt. Puree until smooth.

3. In a large skillet, heat the remaining 2 teaspoons oil over medium heat. Reserving the marinade, lift the shrimp from the bowl, add to the pan, and cook for 1 minute. Turn the shrimp over, add the reserved marinade, and cook for 2 minutes or until the shrimp are opaque.

4. In a large bowl, toss the shrimp with the endives and kiwi. Divide among 4 plates and drizzle the avocado dressing over.

Per serving: 220 calories • 25g protein • 8g fat (1g saturated) • 5g fiber • 13g carbohydrate • 506mg sodium • 22mg magnesium

If you have gluten issues: Choose a gluten-free brand of Greek yogurt.

Cooking for One: In a small bowl, combine 1 tablespoon orange juice, ¾ teaspoon lime juice, and a pinch of salt. Add ¼ pound shrimp and set aside. Make the whole batch of dressing. Cook the shrimp in ½ teaspoon oil, then add to a bowl and toss with 1 small Belgian endive and ½ kiwi. Dress the salad with 3 tablespoons of the dressing (refrigerate the remainder for other salads).

Shrimp Stir-Fry

Hands-On Time: 25 minutes | **Total Time:** 25 minutes | **Makes:** 4 servings

Bags of shrimp are often sold frozen in supermarkets and are quite economical. Buy a bag, remove the shrimp you need, and pop the rest back in the freezer. Seven large shrimp (about what you'll get per serving in this dish) provide 6½ grams of lean protein for just 35 calories! And as a source of omega-3 fats, shrimp will cool inflammation while you lose weight.

1⅓ cups water

⅔ cup quick-cooking brown rice

1 tablespoon plus 1 teaspoon extra-virgin olive oil

¼ cup finely chopped fresh ginger

3 cups sliced bok choy

2 heads Belgian endive, halved lengthwise and cut crosswise into ½-inch-wide slices

½ teaspoon salt

1 pound large shrimp, peeled and deveined

½ cup canned sliced water chestnuts

2 teaspoons sesame oil

1 teaspoon sesame seeds

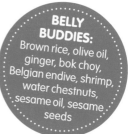

BELLY BUDDIES: Brown rice, olive oil, ginger, bok choy, Belgian endive, shrimp, water chestnuts, sesame oil, sesame seeds

1. In a medium saucepan, bring the water to a boil over high heat. Add the rice and cook according to package directions.

2. Meanwhile, in a large nonstick skillet, heat the olive oil over medium heat. Add the ginger and cook, stirring occasionally, for 2 minutes, or until tender. Add the bok choy, endive, and salt and cook, stirring occasionally, for 4 minutes, or until crisp-tender.

3. Add the shrimp and water chestnuts and drizzle with the sesame oil. Cook, tossing the shrimp occasionally, for 3 minutes, or until opaque throughout.

4. Serve the stir-fry over the rice and sprinkle with the sesame seeds.

Per serving: 252 calories • 24g protein • 11g fat (1g saturated) • 3.5g fiber • 17g carbohydrate • 573mg sodium • 21mg magnesium

Cooking for One: In a small saucepan, cook 3 tablespoons rice according to package directions. In a small skillet, cook 1 tablespoon chopped ginger in 1 teaspoon olive oil until tender. Add ¾ cup sliced bok choy, ½ head sliced Belgian endive, and ⅛ teaspoon salt and cook until crisp-tender. Add ¼ pound shrimp, 2 tablespoons sliced water chestnuts, and ½ teaspoon sesame oil, and cook, tossing the shrimp occasionally, for 2 to 3 minutes, or until opaque throughout. Serve over rice and sprinkle with ¼ teaspoon sesame seeds.

Scallop Hotpot with Rice Noodles

Hands-On Time: 25 minutes | **Total Time:** 30 minutes | **Makes:** 4 servings

A hotpot is a traditional Chinese dish where ingredients are added to a simmering pot of broth and usually cooked tableside. We've taken a little liberty and cooked it in the kitchen. Vegetables and scallops are simmered in light coconut milk, which makes this creamy, yet easy on your digestive system. Snow peas contain some FODMAPs, but the small amount used in this recipe adds a little crunch without any tummy troubles

BELLY BUDDIES: Coconut milk, cucumber, tomato, scallops

- 1 cup light coconut milk
- 1 tablespoon cornstarch
- ½ cup fresh basil leaves, coarsely chopped
- ¼ teaspoon salt
- ⅛ teaspoon cayenne pepper
- 20 snow pea pods, strings removed, halved crosswise
- 1 teaspoon grated lime zest
- 1 tablespoon fresh lime juice
- ¼ cup chopped fresh cilantro

- 2 Kirby cucumbers or 1 regular cucumber, halved lengthwise, seeded, and thinly sliced crosswise lengthwise, seeded and thinly sliced crosswise
- 1 plum tomato, diced
- 1 pound sea scallops, halved horizontally
- 4 ounces thin brown rice noodles

1. In a large skillet, combine the coconut milk, cornstarch, basil, salt, and cayenne and bring to a simmer over low heat. Add the snow peas, cucumbers, tomato, and scallops. Cover and cook for 5 minutes, or until the scallops are just opaque throughout. Remove from the heat and stir in the lime zest and juice and cilantro.

2. Meanwhile, cook the rice noodles according to package directions. Drain.

3. Divide the rice noodles among 4 serving bowls and spoon on the scallops and sauce.

Per serving: 306 calories • 30g protein • 4.5g fat (2.5g saturated) • 3.5g fiber • 35g carbohydrate • 496mg sodium • 15mg magnesium

Cooking for One: In a small skillet, heat ¼ cup light coconut milk, ¾ teaspoon cornstarch, 2 tablespoons basil, and a pinch each of salt and cayenne. Add 5 snow peas, ½ kirby cucumber, 3 tablespoons diced tomato, ¼ pound sea scallops, and ¼ teaspoon grated lime zest. Cook for 3 to 5 minutes, or until the scallops are done. Add 1 tablespoon chopped cilantro. Cook 1 ounce of rice noodles according to package directions and drain. Serve the scallops and sauce on top of the noodles.

Tofu Coconut Curry

Hands-On Time: 25 minutes | **Total Time:** 40 minutes | **Makes:** 4 (2½-cup) servings

Check the label on the curry powder to make certain it doesn't contain either onion or garlic, and to see whether it's mild, medium, or hot. The neutral flavors of tofu and coconut milk will stand up well to a fair amount of curry powder, even the hot type. Tofu is a great low-FODMAP source of vegan protein.

⅓ cup quick-cooking brown rice

2 teaspoons extra-virgin olive oil

¼ cup finely chopped fresh ginger

1 tablespoon curry powder (look for brands with no onions or garlic)

1 cup water

½ pound sweet potato, peeled and cut into ½-inch chunks

½ pound green beans, cut into 1-inch lengths

½ pound plum tomatoes, coarsely chopped

¾ teaspoon salt

1 cup light coconut milk

2 containers (14 ounces each) extra-firm tofu, drained and cut into 1-inch chunks

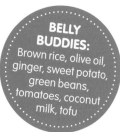

BELLY BUDDIES: Brown rice, olive oil, ginger, sweet potato, green beans, tomatoes, coconut milk, tofu

1. Cook the brown rice according to package directions.

2. In a large saucepan, heat the oil over medium-low heat. Add the ginger and cook for 1 minute, or until tender. Stir in the curry powder and cook for 1 minute.

3. Add the water, sweet potato, green beans, tomatoes, and salt and simmer for 10 minutes, or until the vegetables are tender.

4. Add the coconut milk and tofu and simmer for 3 minutes, or until the tofu is heated through. Stir in the rice and serve.

Per serving: 358 calories • 23g protein • 16g fat (4g saturated) • 7.5g fiber • 32g carbohydrate • 487mg sodium • 37mg magnesium

If you have gluten issues: Choose a gluten-free brand of curry powder.

Fettuccine "Alfredo"

Hands-On Time: 15 minutes I **Total Time:** 25 minutes I **Makes:** 4 servings

In this mock Alfredo, pureed tofu stands in for the heavy cream usually found in this classic Italian pasta dish and green beans masquerade as green peas (you can dice them, if you like, to be the same size as peas). Serve the pasta with a tossed salad, such as Crisp Green Salad with Nuts in a Ginger Dressing (page 217).

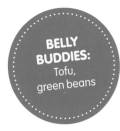

BELLY BUDDIES: Tofu, green beans

7 ounces firm tofu

½ cup lactose-free 1% milk

¼ teaspoon black pepper

¼ cup diced dry-pack sun-dried tomatoes

1¼ teaspoons salt

8 ounces brown rice fettuccine

½ pound green beans

½ cup grated Parmesan cheese

1. In a blender, puree the tofu and milk (it will have the consistency of thick heavy cream). Transfer to a saucepan and add the pepper, sun-dried tomatoes, and ¼ teaspoon of the salt and bring to a simmer. Simmer gently for 2 minutes, then remove from the heat and cover to keep warm.

2. Bring a large pot of water to a boil. Add the pasta and the remaining 1 teaspoon salt and cook according to package directions. Add the beans for the last 3 minutes of cook time.

Reserving 1 cup of the cooking water, drain and return to the pot.

3. Add the tofu sauce, cheese, and ½ cup of the reserved pasta cooking water, tossing to coat evenly. Add more pasta water, if necessary, to loosen up the sauce.

Per serving: 336 calories • 15g protein • 6g fat (2.5g saturated) • 3.5g fiber • 52g carbohydrate • 386mg sodium • 29mg magnesium

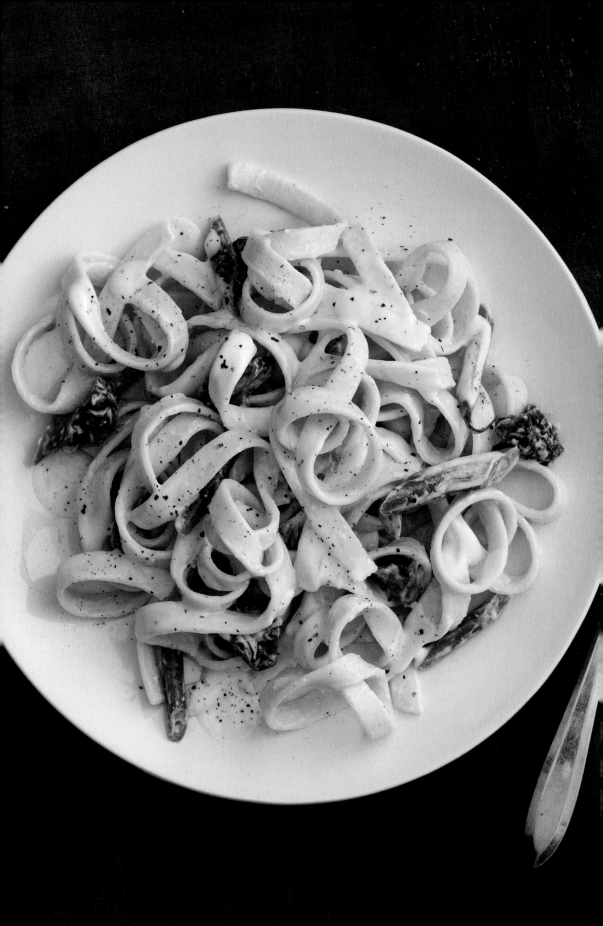

Savory Vegetable Kugel

Hands-On Time: 10 minutes | **Total Time:** 50 minutes plus standing time | **Makes:** 4 servings

A kugel is a traditional Jewish vegetarian casserole usually made with egg noodles. Here we've substituted gluten-free noodles, which are less carb-dense, and pumped up the greens. Arugula provides omega-3 fatty acids, while spinach boosts magnesium intake, both of which fight inflammation. If you have extra greens, make a crisp side salad to go with this dish. If you want to serve this as a side dish, just cut the pan into 8 servings instead of 4 and serve alongside Grilled Chicken with Salsa Verde (page 136).

BELLY BUDDIES: Olive oil, bell pepper, eggs, spinach/arugula

Olive oil cooking spray

2 teaspoons extra-virgin olive oil

1 large red bell pepper, diced

8 ounces brown rice tagliatelle or other short, flat noodles

1 teaspoon salt

3 large eggs

2 large egg whites

¼ cup lactose-free 1% milk

¼ teaspoon black pepper

Large pinch of grated nutmeg

3 cups packed baby spinach, arugula, or a combination of the two (about 3 ounces)

¾ cup shredded part-skim mozzarella

¼ cup grated Parmesan cheese

1. Preheat the oven to 350°F. Line an 8 x 8-inch baking pan with foil (for easier cleanup) and coat the foil with cooking spray.

2. In a medium nonstick skillet, heat the oil over medium-high heat. Add the bell pepper and cook for 3 minutes, or until just beginning to soften. Let cool.

3. Meanwhile, in a large pot of boiling water, add the noodles and ¾ teaspoon of the salt. Cook until 2 minutes shy of the time given in the package directions. Drain.

4. In a large bowl, whisk together the whole eggs, egg whites, milk, pepper, nutmeg, and the remaining ¼ teaspoon salt. Stir in the sautéed bell pepper, spinach, mozzarella, and drained noodles.

5. Transfer the mixture to the baking pan. Cover with foil and bake for 25 minutes. Uncover, sprinkle with the Parmesan, and bake for 10 minutes, or until the cheese has melted and is beginning to brown. Let stand for at least 10 minutes before cutting into 4 servings.

Per serving: 411 calories • 20g protein • 12g fat (4g saturated) • 3g fiber • 49g carbohydrate • 541mg sodium • 16mg magnesium

Tofu Tabbouleh

Hands-On Time: 15 minutes | **Total Time:** 45 minutes plus cooling time |
Makes: 4 (1¾-cup) servings

If you have the time, let the tofu drain on paper towels for a bit before baking. Do this before you cut it into cubes, when it's still in two slabs. Then be sure to check the baked tofu at about 20 minutes instead of 25, since it may bake more quickly.

1 container (14 ounces) extra-firm tofu

½ teaspoon ground cumin

½ teaspoon turmeric

¼ teaspoon black pepper

2 teaspoons plus 2 tablespoons extra-virgin olive oil

¾ teaspoon coarse (kosher) salt

¾ cup brown rice couscous

3 tablespoons fresh lemon juice

1 cup chopped fresh mint

1 pint grape tomatoes, quartered

3 mini cucumbers, quartered lengthwise and cut crosswise into small chunks

Lemon wedges

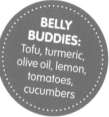

BELLY BUDDIES: Tofu, turmeric, olive oil, lemon, tomatoes, cucumbers

1. Preheat the oven to 400°F. Line a baking sheet with parchment paper.

2. Halve the block of tofu horizontally, then cut each slab into 20 cubes (for a total of 40). In a large bowl, toss the tofu with the cumin, turmeric, pepper, and 2 teaspoons of the oil. Spread on the baking sheet and roast for 25 to 30 minutes, or until firm and beginning to brown. Remove from the oven, return to the same bowl, sprinkle with ½ teaspoon of the salt, toss to coat, and let cool to room temperature.

3. Meanwhile, in a saucepan, cook the couscous according to package directions, with the remaining ¼ teaspoon salt. Fluff with a fork.

4. In a small bowl, whisk together the lemon juice and remaining 2 tablespoons oil.

5. In a salad bowl, combine the cooked couscous, lemon dressing, mint, tomatoes, and cucumbers and toss gently to combine. Add the tofu cubes and toss again.

6. Serve with lemon wedges for squeezing.

Per serving: 338 calories • 14g protein • 16g fat (2g saturated) • 6.5g fiber • 39g carbohydrate • 373mg sodium • 26mg magnesium

Cooking for One: Leftovers of this salad will hold up well in the refrigerator for at least 5 days.

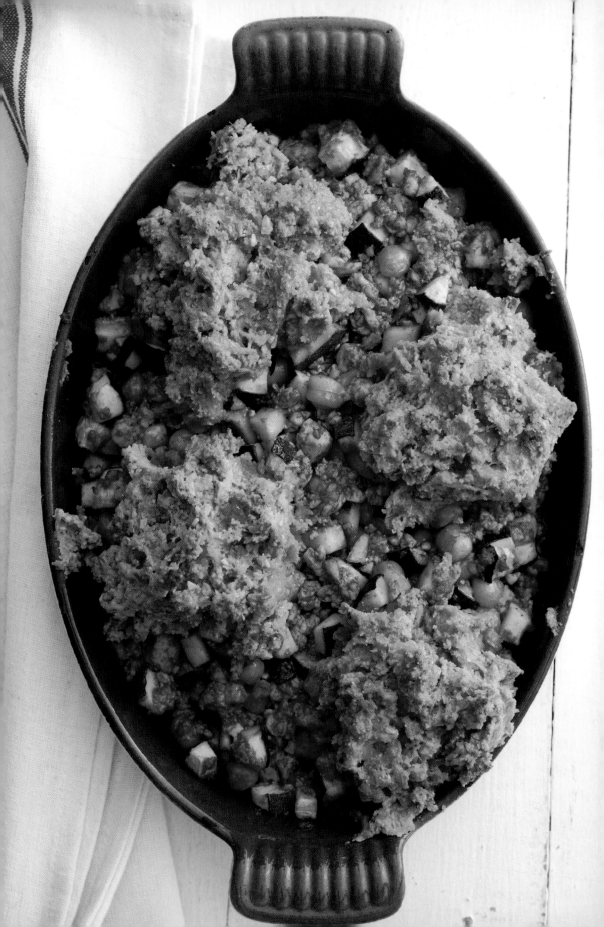

Vegetarian Tamale Pie

Hands-On Time: 20 minutes | **Total Time:** 1 hour 15 minutes | **Makes:** 4 servings

You can find masa harina, a type of Mexican corn flour, in the ethnic section of the supermarket. Tamale dough is typically made with lard, but we used olive oil, a healthier fat. The dough also gets healthy fats from pumpkin seeds, which also provide your body with anti-inflammatory magnesium.

4 teaspoons extra-virgin olive oil

1 container (14 ounces) extra-firm tofu, drained and coarsely chopped

1 tablespoon plus 1 teaspoon chili powder (look for brands with no onions or garlic)

½ teaspoon salt

¼ cup no-salt-added tomato paste (look for brands with no onions or garlic)

3 tablespoons plus ⅔ cup water

1 large zucchini (10 ounces), very finely chopped

½ cup canned no-salt-added chickpeas, drained, rinsed, and coarsely chopped

¾ cup masa harina

¼ cup Parmesan cheese

¼ cup hulled pumpkin seeds (pepitas), finely chopped

1 teaspoon baking powder

1 large egg, lightly beaten

Olive oil cooking spray

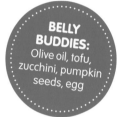

BELLY BUDDIES: Olive oil, tofu, zucchini, pumpkin seeds, egg

1. Preheat the oven to 375°F.

2. In a large nonstick skillet, heat 2 teaspoons of the oil over medium-high heat. Add the tofu and sprinkle with 1 tablespoon of the chili powder and ¼ teaspoon of the salt. Cook the tofu, breaking it up into fine crumbles, for 5 minutes to firm up slightly. Stir in the tomato paste and 3 tablespoons water, stirring until well combined.

3. Remove from the heat and add the zucchini and chickpeas, tossing to combine. Scrape the mixture into an 8 x 8-inch baking pan.

4. In a small bowl, stir together the masa harina, cheese, pumpkin seeds, baking powder, and the remaining 1 teaspoon chili powder and ¼ teaspoon salt. Stir in the egg and the remaining 2 teaspoons oil and ⅔ cup water.

5. Dollop the dough over the top of the filling and spread the dough evenly. Coat the top lightly with cooking spray. Bake for 35 to 45 minutes, or until the top is lightly browned. Remove from the oven, cover with foil, and let stand for 10 minutes.

Per serving: 378 calories • 22g protein • 19g fat (3.5g saturated) • 7g fiber • 33g carbohydrate • 594mg sodium • 85mg magnesium

If you have gluten issues: Choose gluten-free brands of chili powder and baking powder.

Avocado, Tomato, Spinach & Sprout Salad

Chapter 8
Salads

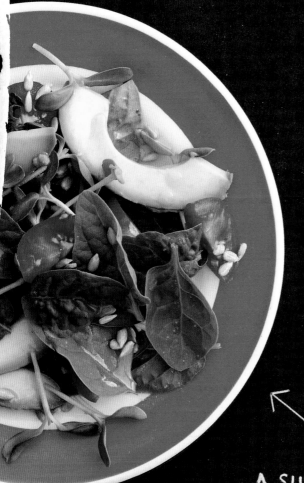

ROUND OUT YOUR MEALS WHILE WHITTLING DOWN YOUR WAISTLINE

A SUPER MAGNESIUM SOURCE

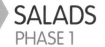
Arugula Salad with Pine Nuts and Parmesan

Hands-On Time: 10 minutes | **Total Time:** 10 minutes | **Makes:** 4 (1¼-cup) servings

Baby arugula has less of a bite than regular but is still pungent enough to stand up to the lemony dressing. The bits of lemon are a nice touch, but feel free to omit them for a mellower salad. Arugula is one of the few plant sources of omega-3 fats, which are linked with lowering the risk of Alzheimer's disease and depression, in addition to reducing the inflammation that can bother your belly.

BELLY BUDDIES:
Lemon, olive oil, arugula, pine nuts

1 lemon plus 4 teaspoons lemon juice

2 tablespoons extra-virgin olive oil

½ teaspoon salt

6 cups baby arugula (6 ounces)

2 teaspoons toasted pine nuts

1 ounce Parmesan cheese, shaved with a vegetable peeler

1. Cut off a thin slice from both ends of the lemon and set it upright on a work surface. Following the curve of the fruit, use a sharp knife to cut off the peel and the membrane surrounding the fruit. With the knife, cut in between the sections of the lemon to release the segments from the membranes. Remove any seeds and cut the lemon segments into ¼-inch bits.

2. In a medium bowl, whisk together the oil, lemon juice, and salt. Add the arugula, lemon bits, and pine nuts and toss to coat.

3. Divide among 4 salad plates and top with the Parmesan.

Per serving: 114 calories • 4g protein • 10g fat (2g saturated) • 2g fiber • 5g carbohydrate • 417mg sodium • 30mg magnesium

Cooking for One: Omit the whole lemon. Make a dressing with 1 teaspoon lemon juice, 1½ teaspoons olive oil, and ⅛ teaspoon salt. Add 1½ cups arugula, ½ teaspoon pine nuts, and 1½ teaspoons Parmesan.

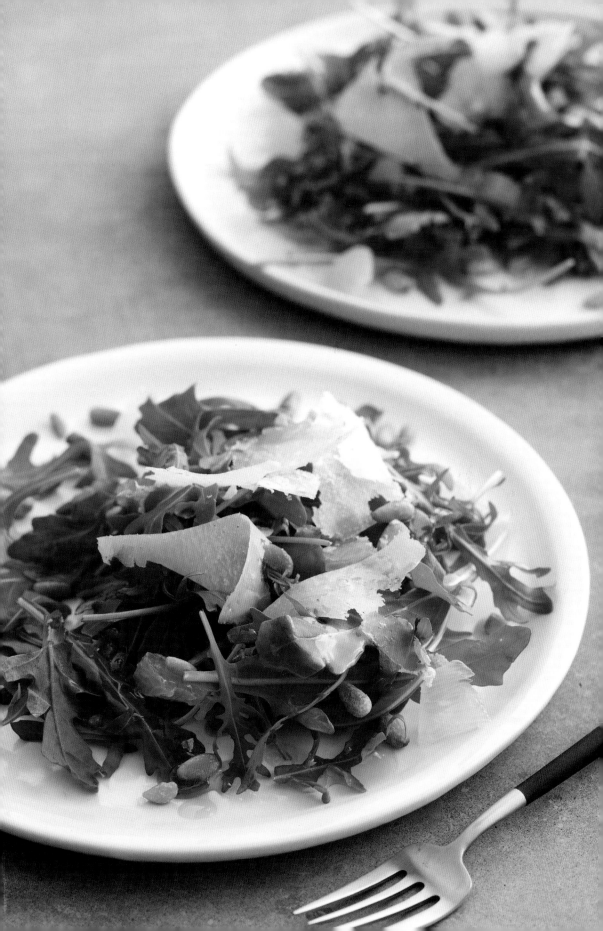

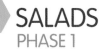
Honeymoon Salad with Green Goddess Dressing

Hands-On Time: 15 minutes | **Total Time:** 15 minutes | **Makes:** 4 (1½-cup) servings

"Honeymoon salad" is diner talk for a salad that is lettuce alone (or "let us alone"). We've paired it with a savory green goddess dressing. Anchovies add a slightly salty richness to the dressing. You won't be using a whole jar or tin of anchovies, but luckily they'll keep in the oil they were packed in for a few months in the refrigerator. If they came in a tin, transfer them to a glass container. You can use anchovies when sautéing vegetables: Finely chop one or two and add them to the oil that you're using; they'll melt down and add great flavor. Or, chop one or two and add to your favorite tomato sauce for pasta.

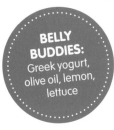

BELLY BUDDIES:
Greek yogurt, olive oil, lemon, lettuce

½ cup packed fresh basil leaves

1 tablespoon snipped chives or sliced scallion greens

4 anchovy fillets, rinsed

½ cup nonfat plain Greek yogurt

1 tablespoon plus 1 teaspoon extra-virgin olive oil

1 tablespoon fresh lemon juice

6 cups sliced romaine lettuce

1. In a blender, combine the basil, chives, anchovies, yogurt, oil, and lemon juice and puree until smooth.

2. Transfer the dressing to a large bowl. Add the lettuce and toss to coat.

Per serving: 74 calories • 4g protein • 5g fat (0.5g saturated) • 1.5g fiber • 4g carbohydrate • 147mg sodium • 14mg magnesium

If you have gluten issues: Choose a gluten-free brand of Greek yogurt.

Cooking for One: Make the whole batch of dressing and store in the refrigerator. For a single portion of salad, toss 1½ cups sliced romaine lettuce with 2½ tablespoons of the dressing.

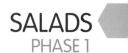

Crisp Green Salad with Nuts in a Ginger Dressing

Hands-On Time: 15 minutes | **Total Time:** 15 minutes | **Makes:** 4 (1¼-cup) servings

The spiciness of fresh ginger in the dressing is balanced by sweet maple syrup, tart lemon juice, and mild, briny tamari. For an easy change of pace, swap in chopped walnuts for the almonds and hulled pumpkin seeds for the sunflower seeds. Tamari is a naturally brewed form of soy sauce; we chose the reduced-sodium version to chop off about 300 milligrams of belly-bloating sodium per tablespoon.

> **BELLY BUDDIES:** Ginger, lemon, maple syrup, olive oil, lettuce, almonds, sunflower seeds

- 1 piece (about 3 inches) fresh ginger (no need to peel)
- 2 teaspoons reduced-sodium tamari or soy sauce
- 1½ teaspoons fresh lemon juice
- 1 teaspoon maple syrup
- ¼ teaspoon salt

- 1 tablespoon extra-virgin olive oil
- 5 cups sliced romaine lettuce
- 3 tablespoons sliced almonds
- 2 teaspoons hulled sunflower seeds

1. Grate the ginger into a small bowl. With your fingers, squeeze the ginger to extract 1 tablespoon juice (grate a little more ginger if necessary). Discard the ginger pulp. Whisk the tamari, lemon juice, maple syrup, and salt into the ginger juice. Then whisk in the oil.

2. In a large bowl, combine the lettuce, almonds, and sunflower seeds and toss to combine. Add the dressing and toss again.

Per serving: 82 calories • 2g protein • 6.5g fat (0.5g saturated) • 2g fiber • 5g carbohydrate • 267mg sodium • 26mg magnesium

If you have gluten issues: Choose a gluten-free brand of tamari.

Cooking for One: Make the full batch of dressing and refrigerate. For a single portion of salad, toss together 1¼ cups sliced romaine, 2 teaspoons sliced almonds, and ½ teaspoon sunflower seeds. Toss with 2 teaspoons of the dressing.

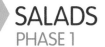

Avocado, Tomato, Spinach, and Sprout Salad

Hands-On Time: 25 minutes | **Total Time:** 25 minutes | **Makes:** 4 (2¼-cup) servings

Choose creamy Hass avocados for this simple salad. You can turn it into a main dish by adding cooked chicken breast or shrimp (about 5 ounces per person). Avocado is rich in belly-trimming monounsaturated fats but is relatively high in calories and FODMAPs, so we've limited the amount here.

BELLY BUDDIES:
Olive oil, lemon, avocado, tomatoes, spinach, sunflower seeds

1 tablespoon extra-virgin olive oil

2 tablespoons fresh lemon juice

1 teaspoon Dijon mustard (look for brands with no onions or garlic)

½ teaspoon salt

½ avocado, sliced

3 plum tomatoes, sliced

5 ounces baby spinach

1 cup sunflower sprouts

2 teaspoons hulled sunflower seeds

1. In a large bowl, whisk together the oil, lemon juice, mustard, and salt.

2. Add the avocado, tomatoes, spinach, sprouts, and sunflower seeds and toss to combine.

Per serving: 135 calories • 3g protein • 10g fat (1.5g saturated) • 5.5g fiber • 12g carbohydrate • 385mg sodium • 29mg magnesium

If you have gluten issues: Choose a gluten-free brand of mustard.

Cooking for One: Make a dressing with ¾ teaspoon olive oil, 1½ teaspoons lemon juice, ¼ teaspoon Dijon mustard, and ⅛ teaspoon salt. Add ⅛ sliced avocado, 1 sliced tomato, 1¼ cups baby spinach, ¼ cup sunflower sprouts, and ½ teaspoon sunflower seeds and toss to combine.

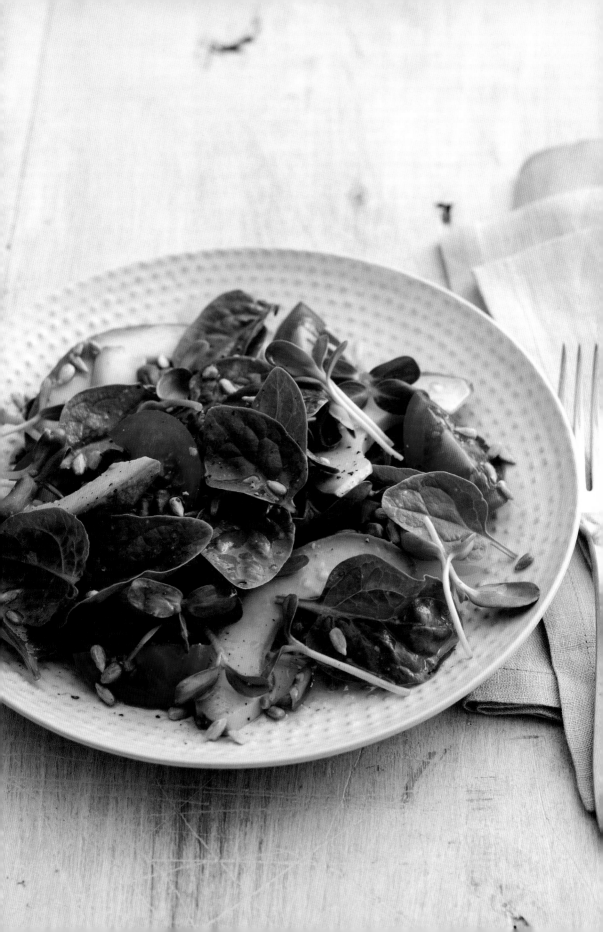

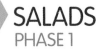

Kiwi and Orange Salad

Hands-On Time: 15 minutes | **Total Time:** 15 minutes | **Makes:** 4 servings

Juicy and sweet, one orange provides more than 100 percent of your daily vitamin C needs plus 3.5 grams of fiber! Having too little vitamin C in the blood stream is linked with bigger waistlines and increased body fat (no thanks!). And, of course, fiber keeps us full and our digestive tract moving. For a nice color contrast, use red-fleshed blood oranges (fall and winter) or cara cara oranges (late summer into the fall). When gold kiwifruit are in season (late spring through early fall), try them in place of the green kiwi. This refreshing salad makes a sensational first course or side dish for Jerk Shrimp (page 153).

BELLY BUDDIES: Oranges, lettuce, kiwifruit

2 navel oranges

¼ cup olive oil mayonnaise (look for brands with no onions or garlic)

Pinch of ground allspice

Pinch of black pepper

1 small head Boston lettuce, torn into bite-size pieces

3 kiwifruit, peeled and thinly sliced

1. Cut a small slice off both ends of 1 orange, enough to expose the fruit. Set the orange on end and, following the curve of the fruit, use a sharp knife to cut off the peel. Set a sieve over a bowl. Working over the sieve, use the sharp knife to cut either side of the orange segments to release them from the membranes. When all of the segments are cut out, squeeze the juice from the membranes into the bowl. Repeat with the other orange. Set the segments aside.

2. Whisk the mayonnaise, allspice, and pepper into the orange juice in the bowl.

3. In a large bowl, toss the lettuce with all but ¼ cup of the dressing. Make a bed of lettuce on 4 plates, arrange the orange segments and kiwi slices on top, and drizzle with the reserved dressing.

Per serving: 111 calories • 2g protein • 4.5g fat (0.5g saturated) • 3.5g fiber • 17g carbohydrate • 134mg sodium • 22mg magnesium

Cooking for One: Make a dressing with 1 tablespoon orange juice, 1 tablespoon olive oil mayonnaise, and a very small pinch each of allspice and pepper. Toss half the dressing with 1½ cups cut-up lettuce. Top the lettuce with segments from ½ orange and 1 small sliced kiwi. Drizzle the fruit with the remaining dressing.

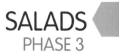
Pickled Bell Pepper Salad

Hands-On Time: 25 minutes | **Total Time:** 25 minutes plus standing time | **Makes:**
6 (generous ½-cup) servings

Serve these quick-pickled peppers as a side salad to any simple grilled
meat, poultry, or fish. They also make a nice side to Tex-Mex Cheeseburgers
(page 130). For fun, bring them to the table in a preserving jar.

½ cup rice vinegar

½ cup water

¼ cup packed light brown sugar

1¼ teaspoons coarse (kosher)
salt

¼ teaspoon black pepper

1 red bell pepper, cut into
½-inch-wide strips

1 yellow bell pepper, cut into
½-inch-wide strips

1 orange bell pepper, cut into
½-inch-wide strips

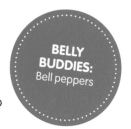

**BELLY
BUDDIES:**
Bell peppers

1. In a medium saucepan, combine
the vinegar, water, brown sugar,
salt, and black pepper and bring to
a boil.

2. Remove from the heat and add
the bell peppers, tossing to coat.
Let them sit for at least 1 hour
before serving warm, at room
temperature, or chilled.

Per serving: 58 calories • 1g protein • 0g fat
(0g saturated) • 1g fiber • 14g carbohydrate •
405mg sodium • 11mg magnesium

Cooking for One: Make the whole
batch. The leftovers hold up well—
they'll keep in the refrigerator for up to
2 weeks.

Cabbage Slaw with Jalapeño-Bacon Dressing

Hands-On Time: 15 minutes | **Total Time:** 15 minutes | **Makes:** 6 (1-cup) servings

Finely shredded raw Brussels sprouts make a delicious addition to a slaw, but if you prefer, just increase the amount of cabbage to 6 cups (about three-quarters of a small head) and omit the Brussels sprouts entirely.

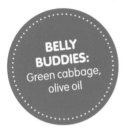

BELLY BUDDIES: Green cabbage, olive oil

- 4 cups shredded green cabbage (½ small head)
- 8 Brussels sprouts, finely shredded
- ½ teaspoon coarse (kosher) salt
- 1 tablespoon plus 2 teaspoons extra-virgin olive oil

- 2 slices uncured Canadian bacon, slivered
- ½ jalapeño pepper, diced
- 3 tablespoons distilled apple cider vinegar

1. In a large bowl, combine the cabbage and Brussels sprouts. Sprinkle with the salt and toss to coat.

2. In a small saucepan, heat the oil over medium-high heat. Add the bacon and jalapeño and cook for 1 minute to infuse the oil with flavor and soften the jalapeño slightly. Add the vinegar and bring to a boil.

3. Pour the hot dressing over the cabbage mixture and toss to coat. Serve at room temperature or chilled.

Per serving: 78 calories • 4g protein • 4.5g fat (1g saturated) • 2.5g fiber • 6g carbohydrate • 263mg sodium • 17mg magnesium

Cooking for One: Make the whole batch and have leftovers for lunch. The slaw holds up very well, though it will get softer as it sits.

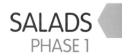

Warm Bok Choy and Pepper Salad

Hands-On Time: 25 minutes | **Total Time:** 25 minutes | **Makes:** 4 (1½-cup) servings

Bok choy is a rich source of vitamin C, beta-carotene, and calcium, which help our digestive enzymes function normally. For the sweetest bok choy, look for young, tender heads. Or if you can find them, use baby bok choy instead. And don't wait until serving an Asian meal; this dish works well with chicken, like Lemon Chicken Under a Brick (page 139), fish and shellfish, such as Jerk Shrimp (page 153), or as part of a vegetarian buffet.

1 tablespoon coconut oil

¼ cup rice vinegar

½ teaspoon ground ginger

½ teaspoon turmeric

½ teaspoon salt

1 tablespoon extra-virgin olive oil

¾ pound bok choy, cut into ½-inch-wide strips

1 red bell pepper, cut into ½-inch-wide strips

1 yellow bell pepper, cut into ½-inch-wide strips

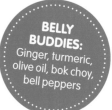

BELLY BUDDIES: Ginger, turmeric, olive oil, bok choy, bell peppers

1. In a large bowl, whisk together the coconut oil, vinegar, ginger, turmeric, and ¼ teaspoon of the salt.

2. In a large nonstick skillet, heat the olive oil over medium heat. Add the bok choy and bell peppers and sprinkle with the remaining ¼ teaspoon salt. Cook, stirring occasionally, for 7 minutes, or until the vegetables are crisp-tender.

3. Scrape the vegetables into the bowl with the dressing and toss to coat. Serve warm or at room temperature.

Per serving: 94 calories • 2g protein • 7g fat (3.5g saturated) • 2g fiber • 7g carbohydrate • 348mg sodium • 26mg magnesium

Cooking for One: Whisk together ¾ teaspoon coconut oil, 1 tablespoon rice vinegar, ⅛ teaspoon each ginger and turmeric, and ⅛ teaspoon salt. Heat ¾ teaspoon olive oil in a small nonstick skillet. Add 1 cup sliced bok choy and ½ cup bell pepper strips. Sprinkle with a pinch of salt and cook until tender. Add to the dressing and toss.

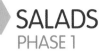

Celery Root Rémoulade with Endives

Hands-On Time: 15 minutes | **Total Time:** 15 minutes plus standing time |
Makes: 6 (1-cup) servings

Celery root, also called celeriac, is a bulblike root vegetable with a crisp texture and a faint celery flavor. In spite of its name, celery root is not actually the root of the celery plant, though the two vegetables are related. This fresh salad of shredded celery root tossed in a rémoulade (creamy mustard dressing) is a typical French bistro dish. The Belgian endives add a nice mild crispness, but you could leave them out and just use a larger celery root. Serve this alongside lean grilled steak, grilled shrimp, or Hazelnut-Stuffed Pork Chops (page 132).

BELLY BUDDIES:
Celery root, lemon, Belgian endives

1 celery root (1¼ pounds), peeled and cut into large chunks

2 teaspoons grated lemon zest

3 tablespoons fresh lemon juice

¾ teaspoon coarse (kosher) salt

¼ cup plus 2 tablespoons olive oil mayonnaise (look for brands with no onions or garlic)

2 teaspoons Dijon mustard (look for brands with no onions or garlic)

2 Belgian endives, thinly sliced crosswise

½ cup chopped flat-leaf parsley

1. In a food processor with a shredding blade, shred the celery root. Transfer to a large bowl and toss with the lemon zest, 2 tablespoons of the lemon juice, and the salt. Set aside for 15 minutes to soften slightly.

2. Meanwhile, in a small bowl, blend together the mayonnaise, mustard, and the remaining 1 tablespoon lemon juice.

3. Add the dressing, endives, and parsley to the celery root mixture and toss to coat.

Per serving: 86 calories • 2g protein • 4.5g fat (0.5g saturated) • 3g fiber • 10g carbohydrate • 495mg sodium • 23mg magnesium

If you have gluten issues: Choose a gluten-free brand of mustard.

Cooking for One: The salad will hold up well, so make the whole batch and store in the refrigerator.

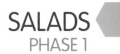

Cucumber, Feta, and Mint Salad

Hands-On Time: 20 minutes | **Total Time:** 20 minutes | **Makes:** 4 (1¾-cup) servings

Peppermint or spearmint, the choice is yours. Peppermint is what you'll generally find in the supermarket, but if you're a fan of strongly flavored mint, look for spearmint in farmers' markets and specialty stores—it is more robust than peppermint.

1 tablespoon plus 1½ teaspoons extra-virgin olive oil

1 tablespoon plus 1½ teaspoons fresh lemon juice

¼ teaspoon salt

⅛ teaspoon cayenne pepper

8 Kirby cucumbers or 4 regular cucumbers, halved lengthwise, seeded, and thinly sliced crosswise

3 ounces reduced-fat feta cheese, crumbled

¼ cup fresh mint leaves, coarsely chopped

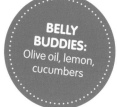

BELLY BUDDIES: Olive oil, lemon, cucumbers

In a large bowl, whisk together the oil, lemon juice, salt, and cayenne. Add the cucumbers, cheese, and mint and toss gently to combine. Serve right away or chill until ready to serve.

Per serving: 103 calories • 6g protein • 8g fat (2.5g saturated) • 1.5g fiber • 4g carbohydrate • 441mg sodium • 4mg magnesium

Cooking for One: Whisk together 1 teaspoon each oil and lemon juice. Add a pinch each of salt and cayenne and fold in 2 thinly sliced Kirby cucumbers, ¾ ounce (about 3 tablespoons) crumbled reduced-fat feta cheese, and 1 tablespoon chopped mint.

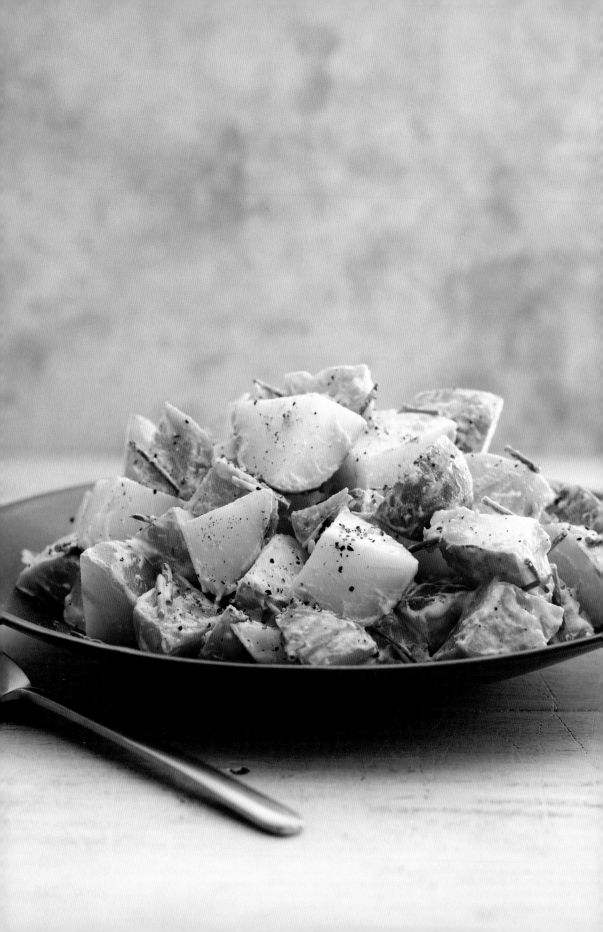

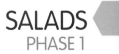

Zesty Orange and White Potato Salad

Hands-On Time: 20 minutes | **Total Time:** 30 minutes | **Makes:** 4 (1-cup) servings

Tossing the potatoes in the tangy yogurt dressing while they're still warm helps them absorb the flavor. If you don't have a large steamer, steam the potatoes in batches.

1 pound red potatoes, well scrubbed and cut into 1-inch chunks

½ pound sweet potatoes, peeled and cut into 1-inch chunks

1 cup nonfat plain Greek yogurt

1 tablespoon extra-virgin olive oil

½ teaspoon salt

1 tablespoon white wine vinegar

2 teaspoons Dijon mustard (look for brands with no onions or garlic)

2 tablespoons snipped chives or sliced scallion greens

Cracked black pepper

BELLY BUDDIES:
Potatoes, sweet potatoes, Greek yogurt, olive oil

1. In a large steamer, steam the red potatoes and sweet potatoes for 10 minutes, or until tender.

2. Meanwhile, in a large bowl, whisk together the yogurt, oil, vinegar, mustard, and salt.

3. Add the still-warm potatoes and chives to the yogurt dressing, and toss gently to coat. Serve warm or at room temperature. Garnish with cracked black pepper, if you'd like.

Per serving: 176 calories • 8g protein • 3.5g fat (0.5g saturated) • 3g fiber • 27g carbohydrate • 404mg sodium • 34mg magnesium

If you have gluten issues: Choose gluten-free brands of Greek yogurt and mustard.

Cooking for One: Steam ¼ pound red potatoes and 2 ounces sweet potatoes. Whisk together ¼ cup yogurt, ¾ teaspoon oil, ¾ teaspoon vinegar, ½ teaspoon Dijon mustard, and ⅛ teaspoon salt. Add the potatoes and 1½ teaspoons chives and toss to combine.

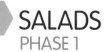
Provençal Eggplant Salad

Hands-On Time: 15 minutes | **Total Time:** 15 minutes plus standing time |
Makes: 4 (1-cup) servings

Fresh eggplant has only 20 calories and about 3 grams of fiber per cup. Plus, it is a source of chlorogenic acid, which may lower your risk of diabetes and weight gain. The method we used to cook the eggplant here is called stir-steaming: It's a cross between steaming and stir-frying, and uses a modest amount of oil. It's a good option for a vegetable like eggplant that sucks up a lot of oil when you sauté it. Serve this alongside broiled or grilled meaty fish, such as tilapia or cod; or get a little fancier and go for the Seared Mahi Mahi with Basil Oil (page 152).

BELLY BUDDIES: Eggplant, olive oil, zucchini, tomatoes, olives

- 1 large eggplant, cut into 1-inch cubes
- ½ teaspoon dried basil
- ½ teaspoon ground fennel
- ¼ teaspoon dried thyme
- ½ teaspoon coarse (kosher) salt
- ¼ cup water
- 3½ teaspoons extra-virgin olive oil

- 1 zucchini (9 ounces), cut into ⅓-inch cubes
- 1 cup quartered grape tomatoes
- ¼ cup chopped kalamata olives
- 1 tablespoon white wine vinegar
- 1 teaspoon Dijon mustard (look for brands with no onions or garlic)

1. In a large nonstick skillet, toss together the eggplant, basil, fennel, thyme, salt, water, and 2 teaspoons of the oil. Cover and bring to a boil over high heat. Reduce the heat to medium and cook for 2 minutes, or until partially tender. Uncover and cook, stirring for 1 minute or until tender and to evaporate some of the remaining liquid.

2. Transfer the eggplant to a salad bowl and stir in the zucchini, tomatoes, and olives.

3. In a small bowl, whisk together the vinegar, mustard, and the remaining 1½ teaspoons oil. Add to the salad and toss well.

4. Let the salad sit for 30 minutes at room temperature (stirring occasionally if you think of it), then refrigerate if making this ahead.

Per serving: 107 calories • 3g protein • 6g fat (1g saturated) • 4.5g fiber • 12g carbohydrate • 370mg sodium • 28mg magnesium

If you have gluten issues: Choose a gluten-free brand of mustard.

Cooking for One: Make the whole batch and refrigerate the leftovers in 1-cup portions for lunches.

Moroccan Carrot Salad

Hands-On Time: 10 minutes | **Total Time:** 30 minutes | **Makes:** 4 (¾-cup) servings

This salad keeps very well in the refrigerator (in fact, the flavors will deepen), so you can make this 1 to 3 days ahead. Choose deep orange carrots for more beta-carotene, which is converted to inflammation-fighting vitamin A in your body. Toss the carrots with Herbed Tricolor Quinoa (page 258) for a satisfying vegetarian meal.

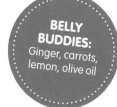

BELLY BUDDIES: Ginger, carrots, lemon, olive oil

¾ teaspoon ground cinnamon
¾ teaspoon ground coriander
¾ teaspoon ground ginger
½ teaspoon salt
⅛ teaspoon cayenne pepper
2 cups water

¾ pound carrots, cut crosswise into ½-inch-thick slices
2 tablespoons fresh lemon juice
1 tablespoon plus 1 teaspoon extra-virgin olive oil
1 teaspoon pure maple syrup

1. In a large skillet, combine the cinnamon, coriander, ginger, salt, cayenne, and water. Bring to a boil over high heat.

2. Add the carrots, reduce to a simmer, cover, and cook for 15 minutes, or until tender.

3. Reserving the cooking liquid, drain the carrots. Measure out ¼ cup of the cooking liquid and transfer to a large bowl. Whisk in the lemon juice, oil, and maple syrup. Add the carrots and toss to coat. Serve at room temperature or chilled.

Per serving: 82 calories • 1g protein • 4.5g fat (0.5g saturated) • 2.5g fiber • 10g carbohydrate • 155mg sodium • 11mg magnesium

Cooking for One: Make the whole batch and refrigerate the leftovers in ¾-cup portions for lunch.

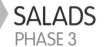

Cherry Tomato and Forbidden Rice Salad

Hands-On Time: 10 minutes | **Total Time:** 55 minutes plus cooling time | **Makes:** 4 (1-cup) servings

Forbidden Rice and Black Japonica are both brand names of a black rice exceptionally rich in anthocyanins, the phytochemicals that make fruits deep red to purple. If you can't find it, just make this with brown rice. To make ginger juice, grate about 3 inches of fresh ginger and then press it in a fine-mesh sieve to extract the juice. You can also buy ginger juice in bottles.

BELLY BUDDIES:
Rice, lime, ginger, olive oil, tomatoes, bell pepper

⅔ cup black rice (Forbidden Rice or Black Japonica)

5 cups water

¾ teaspoon salt

1 teaspoon grated lime zest

3 tablespoons fresh lime juice

2 tablespoons ginger juice

1 tablespoon plus 1 teaspoon extra-virgin olive oil

8 ounces large cherry tomatoes, halved, or small vine-ripened tomatoes, quartered

1 yellow bell pepper, diced

⅓ cup chopped fresh cilantro

1. In a large saucepan, combine the rice, water, and ½ teaspoon of the salt. Bring to a boil over high heat, then reduce to a high simmer, partially cover, and cook for 35 to 45 minutes, or until the rice is tender. Drain well.

2. Meanwhile, in a large bowl, whisk together the lime zest, lime juice, ginger juice, oil, and the remaining ¼ teaspoon salt.

3. Add the warm rice to the dressing in the bowl and toss to combine. Let the rice cool to room temperature.

4. Add the tomatoes, bell pepper, and cilantro. Toss again. Serve at room temperature or chilled.

Per serving: 170 calories • 4g protein • 6g fat (0.5g saturated) • 3g fiber • 29g carbohydrate • 354mg sodium • 55mg magnesium

Cooking for One: Make the whole batch and refrigerate the leftovers in 1-cup portions for lunches.

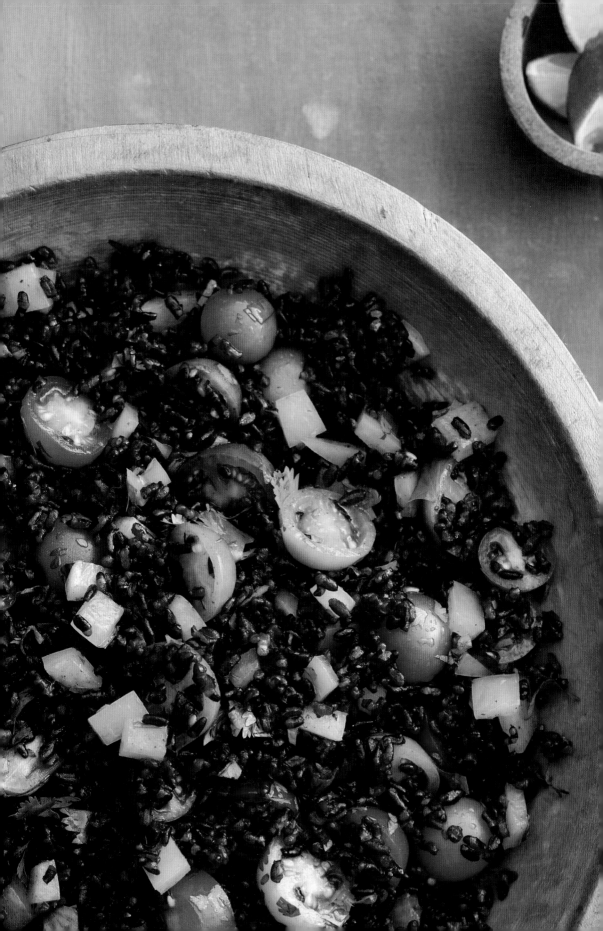

MAPLE-GLAZED CARROTS

Your tummy and your tastebuds will love it!

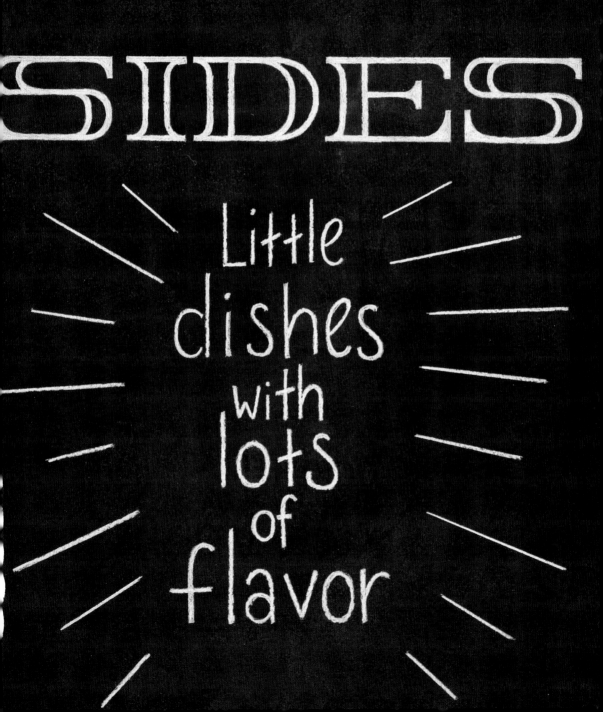

Chapter 9

SIDES

Little dishes with lots of flavor

Grilled Belgian Endives

Hands-On Time: 10 minutes | **Total Time:** 10 minutes | **Makes:** 4 servings

Fresh Belgian endive, which is crisp and mild with a just hint of bitterness, becomes very tender—almost creamy—when cooked. To keep the endive intact when grilling, keep most of the stem on. Simply slice off a thin sliver from the stem end, before halving lengthwise. Serve with Hazelnut-Stuffed Pork Chops (page 132), Barbecue-Glazed Flank Steak (page 129), or Crab Cakes (page 155).

BELLY BUDDIES:
Olive oil,
Belgian endive

1 tablespoon plus 1 teaspoon extra-virgin olive oil

4 Belgian endives (4 ounces each), halved lengthwise

½ teaspoon coarse (kosher) salt

Brush a grill pan with the oil and heat over medium-low heat. Place the endives, cut side down, on the grill pan and cook, turning them as they cook and color, for 3 minutes per side, or until tender. Sprinkle with the salt and serve hot.

Per serving: 59 calories • 1g protein • 4.5g fat (0.5g saturated) • 3.5g fiber • 5g carbohydrate • 242mg sodium • 11mg magnesium

Cooking for One: Grill 1 halved Belgian endive on a grill pan brushed with 1 teaspoon oil. Sprinkle with ⅛ teaspoon salt.

Creamed Kale with Bacon and Hazelnuts

Hands-On Time: 15 minutes | **Total Time:** 45 minutes | **Makes:** 4 (½-cup) servings

To toast the hazelnuts, spread them in a toaster oven tray and bake at 350°F for 3 to 5 minutes, or until fragrant and toasted. Or toast in a dry skillet over medium heat, stirring occasionally, for about the same amount of time. Adding a smattering of nuts is a delicious way to boost magnesium and fiber in your diet.

- 1 teaspoon extra-virgin olive oil
- 2 slices uncured Canadian bacon, coarsely chopped
- 2 cups low-sodium chicken broth (look for brands with no onions or garlic) or Homemade Chicken Broth (page 111)
- 1 bunch kale (1 pound), thick stems discarded and leaves cut crosswise into 1-inch-wide ribbons
- ¼ teaspoon salt
- 4 wedges (¾ ounces each) light spreadable cheese (look for brands with no onions or garlic)
- 2 tablespoons skinned hazelnuts, toasted and chopped

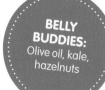

BELLY BUDDIES: Olive oil, kale, hazelnuts

1. In a large nonstick saucepan or Dutch oven, heat the oil over medium-high heat. Add the bacon and cook for 2 to 3 minutes, or until it crisps. With a slotted spoon, transfer the bacon to a plate.

2. Add the broth, kale, and salt to the pan. Cover, reduce the heat to medium, and cook for 25 to 30 minutes, or until the kale is very tender. Stir it down every once in awhile.

3. Transfer the kale and any cooking liquid to a food processor. Add the cheese and puree until it's as smooth as you can get it. (If necessary, add a little water to help with the pureeing.)

4. Serve the kale topped with the bacon and hazelnuts.

Per serving: 122 calories • 8g protein • 6.5g fat (1.5g saturated) • 2.5g fiber • 9g carbohydrate • 541mg sodium • 27mg magnesium

If you have gluten issues: Choose gluten-free brands of chicken broth and light spreadable cheese.

Cooking for One: Make the whole batch and freeze the leftovers in ½-cup portions. Stir the bacon into the puree before freezing but store the hazelnuts in the refrigerator (or toast them fresh when you're ready to serve the leftovers).

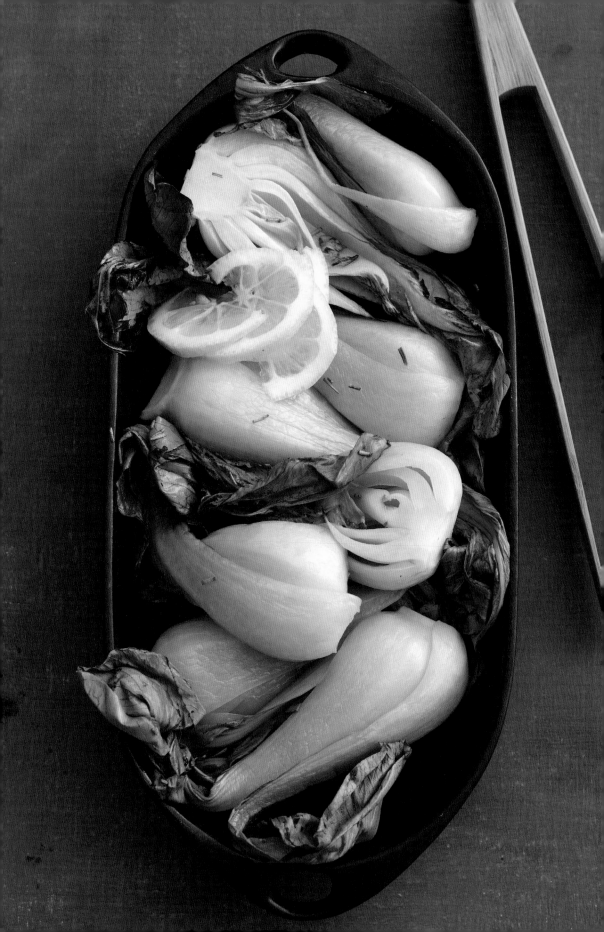

Lemony Roasted Bok Choy

Hands-On Time: 5 minutes | **Total Time:** 35 minutes | **Makes:** 4 (1-cup) servings

Bok choy, sometimes also sold as Chinese cabbage, is crisp and mild in flavor. Baby bok choy are small and tender, but if you can't find them, look for small, mature bok choy that have white, not yellow leaves, without any rust spots.

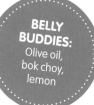

BELLY BUDDIES:
Olive oil, bok choy, lemon

- 1 tablespoon plus 1 teaspoon Roasted Garlic Oil (page 54) or extra-virgin olive oil
- 1 pound baby bok choy
- ½ teaspoon crumbled dried rosemary
- ¾ teaspoon coarse (kosher) salt
- 1 tablespoon plus 1 teaspoon fresh lemon juice

1. Preheat the oven to 375°F.

2. Place the oil in a 9 x 13-inch baking pan. Add the bok choy, rosemary, and salt and toss to coat.

3. Roast, turning the bok choy twice, for 25 to 30 minutes, or until tender and lightly browned. Sprinkle on the lemon juice and toss to coat.

Per serving: 59 calories • 2g protein • 5g fat (0.5g saturated) • 1g fiber • 4g carbohydrate • 434mg sodium • 23mg magnesium

Cooking for One: In a small baking dish or ovenproof skillet, toss ¼ pound bok choy with ⅛ teaspoon dried rosemary, a scant ¼ teaspoon salt, and 1 teaspoon Roasted Garlic Oil (or olive oil) and roast as directed. Toss with 1 teaspoon lemon juice.

Tuscan Green Beans

Hands-On Time: 15 minutes | **Total Time:** 35 minutes | **Makes:** 4 (1-cup) servings

Fresh tomatoes, bright orange zest, and oregano give the green beans an Italian flair. Unlike many green bean recipes, this one calls for cooking the beans beyond crisp-tender, until they are meltingly tender.

BELLY BUDDIES:
Olive oil, green beans, tomatoes

1 tablespoon plus 1 teaspoon Roasted Garlic Oil (page 54) or extra-virgin olive oil

1½ pounds green beans, halved crosswise

¾ pound plum tomatoes, coarsely chopped (1½ cups)

⅓ cup packed fresh basil leaves, coarsely chopped

1 teaspoon grated orange zest

½ teaspoon dried oregano

½ teaspoon salt

In a large skillet, heat the oil over medium heat. Add the green beans, tossing to coat. Add the tomatoes, basil, orange zest, oregano, and salt and bring to a simmer. Cover and cook, stirring once or twice, for 20 minutes, or until the green beans are very tender (the color will not be bright green).

Per serving: 109 calories • 4g protein • 5g fat (0.5g saturated) • 6g fiber • 15g carbohydrate • 305mg sodium • 55mg magnesium

Cooking for One: In a small skillet, heat 1 teaspoon Roasted Garlic Oil (or olive oil) over medium-low heat. Add 6 ounces green beans, tossing to coat. Add 1 small plum tomato (chopped), 1½ tablespoons chopped basil, ¼ teaspoon orange zest, and ⅛ teaspoon each oregano and salt. Cover and cook until very tender.

Sesame-Ginger Green Beans

Hands-On Time: 30 minutes | **Total Time:** 30 minutes | **Makes:** 4 (¾-cup) servings

If you like, give this dish a boost of extra magnesium, fiber, and flavor by sprinkling a teaspoon of sesame seeds over the top once the beans have cooked. To keep them at their freshest, store sesame seeds in the freezer.

2 teaspoons extra-virgin olive oil

1 piece (about 2 inches) fresh ginger, peeled, thinly sliced, and cut into matchsticks (¼ cup)

¾ pound green beans

1 tablespoon plus 1 teaspoon reduced-sodium tamari or soy sauce

⅓ cup water

2 teaspoons sesame oil

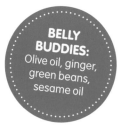

BELLY BUDDIES:
Olive oil, ginger, green beans, sesame oil

1. In a large nonstick skillet, heat the olive oil over medium heat. Add the ginger and cook for 2 minutes.

2. Add the green beans, tamari, and water and bring to a boil. Reduce to a simmer, cover, and cook for 5 minutes.

3. Uncover, stir in the sesame oil, and cook for 5 minutes, or until the green beans are tender and most of the liquid has evaporated.

Per serving: 72 calories • 2g protein • 5g fat (0.5g saturated) • 2.5g fiber • 6g carbohydrate • 239mg sodium • 22mg magnesium

If you have gluten issues: Choose gluten-free brands of tamari.

Cooking for One: In a small nonstick skillet, sauté 1 tablespoon ginger in ½ teaspoon olive oil. Add 3 ounces green beans, 1 teaspoon tamari, and 1½ tablespoons water and cook as directed. Drizzle with ½ teaspoon sesame oil at the end.

Pickled Zucchini Spears

Hands-On Time: 10 minutes | **Total Time:** 15 minutes plus cooling time |
Makes: 6 (½-cup) servings

These may remind you of bread-and-butter pickles. You won't believe these sweet and dilly spears only have 30 calories per serving! Serve them along-side Deviled Chicken (page 145).

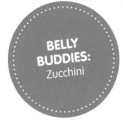

BELLY BUDDIES:
Zucchini

3 medium zucchini (6 ounces each), halved crosswise and quartered lengthwise

¾ teaspoon mustard seeds

½ teaspoon dill seeds

¼ teaspoon red-pepper flakes

¼ cup chopped fresh dill or 6 small sprigs

⅔ cup distilled white vinegar

¼ cup water

1 tablespoon plus 1 teaspoon light brown sugar

¾ teaspoon coarse (kosher) salt

1. Place the zucchini in a bowl along with the mustard seeds, dill seeds, pepper flakes, and fresh dill.

2. In a small saucepan, combine the vinegar, water, brown sugar, and salt and bring to a boil over high heat, stirring to dissolve the sugar. Pour the hot mixture over the zucchini and toss to combine.

3. Let cool to room temperature, then place in a jar or other container and refrigerate for at least 1 day or up to 2 weeks.

Per serving: 30 calories • 1g protein • 0.5g fat (0g saturated) • 1g fiber • 6g carbohydrate • 248mg sodium • 16mg magnesium

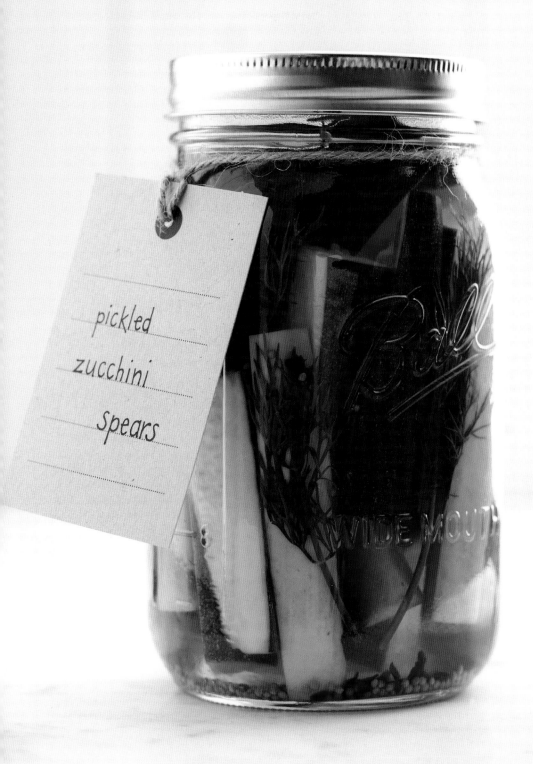

pickled

zucchini

spears

Sautéed Cabbage and Walnuts

Hands-On Time: 10 minutes | **Total Time:** 25 minutes | **Makes:** 4 (¾-cup) servings

Walnuts are tops on our Belly Buddy list. They're low in FODMAPs and high in inflammation-fighting omega-3 fats. This dish makes a nice accompaniment to Maple-Rosemary Roasted Pork Tenderloin (page 133). If you're in Phase 3, you can cook 2 ounces of gluten-free pasta (preferably brown rice or quinoa-corn pasta) and toss it with the finished dish while still hot. Increase the chives to ¼ cup and the chopped dill to ½ cup. Then taste for seasoning—you may need to add a tablespoon more of vinegar.

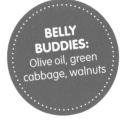

BELLY BUDDIES:
Olive oil, green cabbage, walnuts

1 tablespoon plus 1 teaspoon extra-virgin olive oil

6 cups chunks (1 inch) green cabbage

3 tablespoons snipped chives or sliced scallion greens

½ teaspoon salt

⅓ cup walnuts, chopped

¼ cup chopped fresh dill

1 tablespoon cider vinegar

1. In a large skillet, heat the oil over medium heat. Add the cabbage, chives, and salt and cook, stirring occasionally, for 15 minutes, or until the cabbage is crisp-tender (starting to wilt, but not mushy).

2. Add the walnuts, dill, and vinegar and toss to combine. Serve hot or at room temperature.

Per serving: 121 calories • 3g protein • 10g fat (1g saturated) • 3g fiber • 7g carbohydrate • 260mg sodium • 30mg magnesium

Cooking for One: In a medium skillet, cook 1½ cups cabbage, 2 teaspoons chives, and ⅛ teaspoon salt in 1 teaspoon oil. Add 1 tablespoon dill, ¾ teaspoon vinegar, and a generous tablespoon of chopped walnuts.

Crispy-Topped Broiled Tomatoes

Hands-On Time: 10 minutes | **Total Time:** 15 minutes | **Makes:** 4 servings

Fiber-rich oat bran, rather than carb-dense bread crumbs, makes a crisp topping for sweet, ripe tomatoes. Store oat bran in the freezer where it will stay fresh and keep for several months.

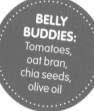

BELLY BUDDIES: Tomatoes, oat bran, chia seeds, olive oil

- 4 beefsteak tomatoes (8 ounces each)
- ½ teaspoon coarse (kosher) salt
- ½ teaspoon crumbled dried rosemary
- ¼ teaspoon black pepper
- 2 tablespoons oat bran
- 1 tablespoon chia seeds
- ⅓ cup grated Parmesan cheese
- 1 tablespoon plus 1 teaspoon extra-virgin olive oil

1. Preheat the broiler with the rack 4 inches from the heat.

2. With a serrated knife, halve the tomatoes horizontally and scoop out a little of the pulp. Place them, cut side up, on a broiler pan. Sprinkle with the salt, rosemary, and pepper and broil for 4 minutes, or until tender.

3. Top each tomato half with ¾ teaspoon oat bran, a scant ¼ teaspoon chia seeds, and a generous 2 teaspoons Parmesan. Drizzle each with ½ teaspoon oil and broil for 1 minute, or until the topping is crisp and browned.

4. Serve 2 tomato halves per person.

Per serving: 130 calories • 6g protein • 8g fat (2g saturated) • 4g fiber • 12g carbohydrate • 354mg sodium • 44mg magnesium

If you have gluten issues: Choose gluten-free brands of oat bran and chia seeds.

Cooking for One: Halve 1 beefsteak tomato horizontally and scoop out a little of the pulp. Sprinkle with ⅛ teaspoon each coarse salt and rosemary, and a pinch of pepper. Broil until tender as directed. Top as directed in step 3 and broil until the topping is crisp.

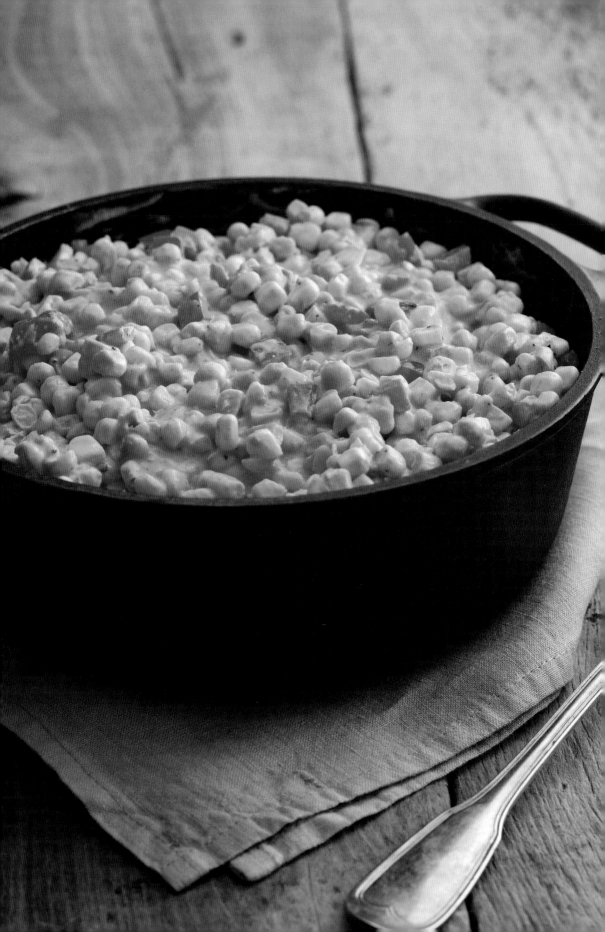

Paprika-Spiced Creamed Corn

Hands-On Time: 10 minutes | **Total Time:** 15 minutes | **Makes:** 4 (½-cup) servings

Smoked paprika comes in both hot and sweet (mild) and can be found on the spice shelf in the supermarket. Check the label and use the one you prefer.

1 teaspoon extra-virgin olive oil
1 red bell pepper, diced
2 teaspoons smoked paprika
3 tablespoons ⅓-less-fat cream cheese (1.5 ounces)

⅔ cup lactose-free 1% milk
2 cups frozen corn kernels
½ teaspoon salt

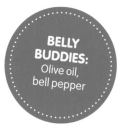

BELLY BUDDIES: Olive oil, bell pepper

1. In a medium saucepan, heat the oil over medium heat. Add the bell pepper and cook, stirring occasionally, for 5 minutes, or until tender. Stir in the paprika and cook for 1 minute.

2. Add the cream cheese and milk and bring to a simmer. Stir in the corn and salt and cook for 5 minutes, or until the corn is heated through and the dish is creamy.

Per serving: 132 calories • 5g protein • 5g fat (2g saturated) • 3g fiber • 20g carbohydrate • 350mg sodium • 35mg magnesium

If you have gluten issues: Choose a gluten-free brand of paprika.

Cooking for One: In a small saucepan, cook ¼ diced bell pepper in ¼ teaspoon oil until tender. Add ½ teaspoon smoked paprika, 2¼ teaspoons cream cheese, 3 tablespoons lactose-free 1% milk, ½ cup corn kernels, and ⅛ teaspoon salt and cook as directed.

Broccoli, Corn, and Grape Tomato Sauté

Hands-On Time: 10 minutes | **Total Time:** 15 minutes | **Makes:** 6 (¾-cup) servings

To save on prep time, buy precut broccoli in the produce department. You'll be amazed how much more often you'll opt for fresh vegetables if you spend just a little extra money for the convenience. You could, of course, make this with frozen broccoli, but it should be well thawed and drained. A 10-ounce package should be the right amount.

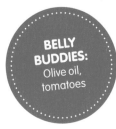

BELLY BUDDIES:
Olive oil, tomatoes

3 cups small broccoli florets (about ½ pound)

4 teaspoons extra-virgin olive oil

1 cup corn kernels (no-salt-added canned or thawed frozen)

1 teaspoon dried tarragon, crumbled

¼ teaspoon black pepper

1 pint grape tomatoes, halved

½ teaspoon salt

1. In a vegetable steamer, cook the broccoli for 3 to 5 minutes, or until bright green and crisp-tender.

2. In a large nonstick skillet, heat the oil over medium-high heat. Add the corn, sprinkle with the tarragon and pepper, and cook for 30 seconds to infuse the oil with a little tarragon flavor.

3. Add the tomatoes, steamed broccoli, and salt and toss to coat. Cook for 3 minutes, or until everything is heated through and the tomatoes are starting to soften.

Per serving: 82 calories • 2g protein • 3.5g fat (0.5g saturated) • 2g fiber • 12g carbohydrate • 204mg sodium • 9mg magnesium

Cooking for One: Make the whole batch and store the leftovers in ¾-cup portions to have as a lunch salad; just stir in a little red wine vinegar to taste. Or to make it a main-dish salad, add 4 ounces cooked diced turkey or chicken breast to a ¾-cup portion.

Herbed Sautéed Radishes

Hands-On Time: 10 minutes | **Total Time:** 10 minutes | **Makes:** 4 (½-cup) servings

You'll be surprised at how sweet and tasty spicy radishes can be when sautéed and sprinkled with a little sugar and vinegar. These can be eaten hot, at room temperature, or chilled. Radishes are low in calories, too—only 18 calories per cup! Serve with Turkey Cutlets in Spicy Peanut Sauce (page 150) or Tandoori-Style Baked Chicken (page 138).

- 1 tablespoon plus 1 teaspoon extra-virgin olive oil
- 1 pound radishes, quartered lengthwise
- 1 tablespoon plus 1 teaspoon light brown sugar
- ½ teaspoon salt
- ¼ cup rice vinegar
- 2 tablespoons chopped fresh tarragon
- 2 tablespoons snipped chives or sliced scallion greens

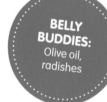

BELLY BUDDIES:
Olive oil, radishes

1. In a large skillet, heat the oil over medium heat. Add the radishes, brown sugar, and salt and cook, tossing frequently, for 5 minutes, or until the radishes are crisp-tender.

2. Add the vinegar and tarragon and cook for 1 minute, or until the liquid is syrupy and the radishes are nicely coated. Garnish with the chives.

Per serving: 77 calories • 1g protein • 4.5g fat (0.5g saturated) • 2g fiber • 9g carbohydrate • 337mg sodium • 14mg magnesium

Cooking for One: Make the whole batch and refrigerate the leftovers in ½-cup portions for lunch.

Grilled Eggplant and Chard Gratin

Hands-On Time: 25 minutes | **Total Time:** 40 minutes | **Makes:** 6 servings

Streamline this recipe by grilling the eggplant and stir-steaming the chard ahead of time. Then the last-minute cooking will only take 15 minutes. Swiss chard is a mild magnesium-rich leafy green that cooks quickly but holds up well in a dish such as a gratin. Pair this dish with grilled chicken breast or flank steak rubbed with cumin, garlic powder, and a little salt.

BELLY BUDDIES: Olive oil, eggplant, Swiss chard, tomatoes

Olive oil cooking spray

1 medium-large eggplant (1 pound), peeled and cut crosswise into ½-inch-thick slices

2 teaspoons extra-virgin olive oil

1 bunch Swiss chard (about 1 pound), stem ends trimmed and stalks and leaves cut crosswise into ½-inch-wide pieces

3 tablespoons water

½ teaspoon salt

5 plum tomatoes, sliced crosswise into ¼-inch-thick slices

¾ cup shredded part-skim mozzarella cheese (3 ounces)

1. Preheat the oven to 350°F. Coat a shallow 1½- to 2-quart baking dish with cooking spray.

2. Preheat a grill pan or cast-iron skillet over medium-high heat. Coat both sides of the eggplant with a little cooking spray. Working in batches, cook the eggplant, flipping once, for 2 to 3 minutes per side, or until semi-tender and grill marks appear.

3. In a large nonstick skillet, heat the oil over medium-high heat. Add the chard, water, and ¼ teaspoon of the salt and toss to coat in the oil. Cover and steam for 4 minutes, or until wilted.

4. Layer the bottom of the baking dish with half the eggplant and sprinkle with ⅛ teaspoon of the salt. Cover with half the chard, half the tomatoes, and ¼ cup of the cheese. Repeat the layering, using the remaining ⅛ teaspoon salt on the eggplant and ending with the remaining ½ cup cheese.

5. Bake for 15 minutes, or until the cheese melts and the vegetables are heated through.

Per serving: 105 calories • 7g protein • 5g fat (1.5g saturated) • 4g fiber • 10g carbohydrate • 459mg sodium • 78mg magnesium

Maple-Orange Grilled Eggplant

Hands-On Time: 10 minutes | **Total Time:** 30 minutes plus standing time |
Makes: 4 servings

We chose baby eggplant because it tends to be sweeter and less seedy than regular eggplant, but there are many varieties in the market. You can choose long, slender Japanese eggplant, small white eggplant, or any firm eggplant.

2 tablespoons fresh orange juice

1 tablespoon plus 2 teaspoons extra-virgin olive oil

2 teaspoons pure maple syrup

1 teaspoon Dijon mustard (look for brands with no onions or garlic)

½ teaspoon salt

Olive oil cooking spray

1½ pounds baby eggplant, cut crosswise into ½-inch-thick rounds

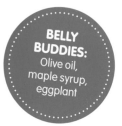

BELLY BUDDIES: Olive oil, maple syrup, eggplant

1. In a shallow bowl, whisk together the orange juice, oil, maple syrup, mustard, and salt.

2. Coat a grill pan with cooking spray and heat over medium-low heat. Add half the eggplant and cook, turning the pieces over, for 10 minutes, or until tender. As the pieces of eggplant are done, add them to the bowl with the maple-orange dressing. Recoat the grill pan and cook the remaining eggplant, adding to the bowl as you go.

3. Turn the eggplant over to coat with the dressing and let stand for 30 minutes before serving.

Per serving: 112 calories • 2g protein • 6.5g fat (1g saturated) • 4.5g fiber • 13g carbohydrate • 325mg sodium • 25mg magnesium

If you have gluten issues: Choose a gluten-free brand of mustard.

Cooking for One: Cook 1 baby eggplant as directed. In a medium bowl, whisk together 1½ teaspoons orange juice, ½ teaspoon maple syrup, ¼ teaspoon mustard, and ⅛ teaspoon salt. Add the eggplant and let stand for 30 minutes.

Maple-Glazed Carrots

Hands-On Time: 15 minutes | **Total Time:** 30 minutes | **Makes:** 4 (½-cup) servings

This is a very simple recipe that you can tinker with to suit your taste. Try adding ¼ teaspoon curry powder or smoked paprika. Try different varieties of carrots for fun. White and yellow carrots have a milder flavor and fewer antioxidants than regular orange carrots, but purple carrots are brimming with good-for-you anthocyanins. Serve the carrots alongside a piece of grilled fish, chicken, or steak.

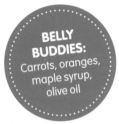

BELLY BUDDIES: Carrots, oranges, maple syrup, olive oil

1 pound carrots (any color), sliced on an angle

3 tablespoons fresh orange juice

1 tablespoon pure maple syrup

1 tablespoon water

2 teaspoons extra-virgin olive oil

½ teaspoon salt

¼ teaspoon black pepper

⅓ cup chopped chives

1. In a medium saucepan, combine the carrots, orange juice, maple syrup, water, oil, salt, and pepper. Bring to a simmer, cover, and cook for 5 minutes.

2. Uncover and stir to coat. Continue cooking, stirring occasionally, for 6 to 8 minutes, or until most of the liquid has evaporated and the carrots are tender and glazed.

3. Stir in the chives and serve hot.

Per serving: 86 calories • 1g protein • 2.5g fat (0.5g saturated) • 3.5g fiber • 16g carbohydrate • 370mg sodium • 18mg magnesium

Cooking for One: These carrots actually make a very nice snack, so make the whole batch and refrigerate the leftovers.

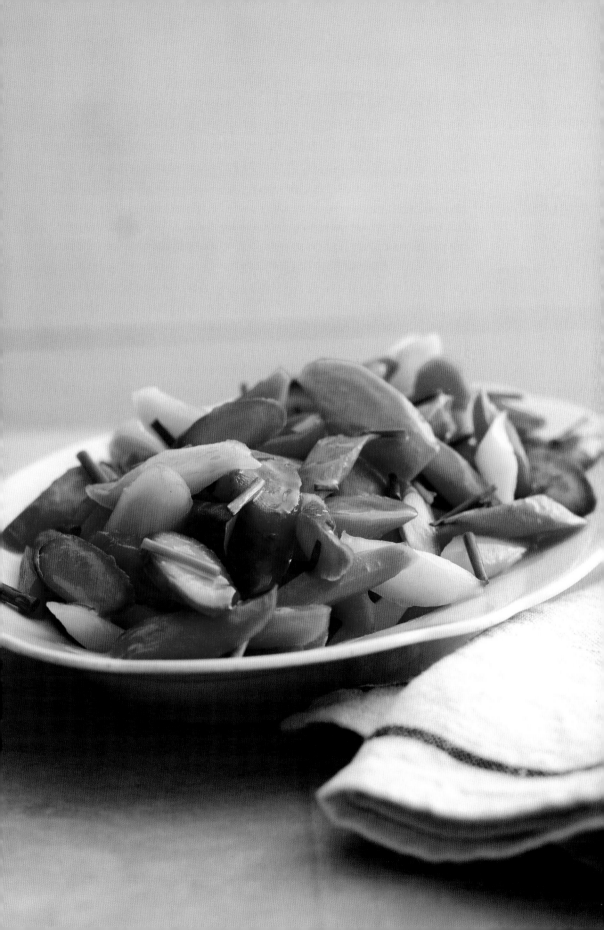

Roasted Parsnips and Carrots

Hands-On Time: 10 minutes | **Total Time:** 40 minutes | **Makes:** 4 (½-cup) servings

If you aren't familiar with parsnips, they are similar in both texture and taste to carrots, but with a slightly spicy flavor. The two work perfectly together, and parsnips can be cooked in many dishes in the same way that carrots can. This dish can be served hot, at room temperature, or chilled. We love the combo of carrots and parsnips in this recipe, which promotes healthy digestion with a whopping 6 grams of fiber.

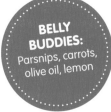

BELLY BUDDIES:
Parsnips, carrots, olive oil, lemon

¾ pound parsnips, peeled
½ pound carrots, peeled
1 tablespoon plus 1 teaspoon extra-virgin olive oil

¾ teaspoon coarse (kosher) salt
1 tablespoon fresh lemon juice

1. Preheat the oven to 400°F.

2. If the parsnips and carrots have thick ends, cut those ends in half lengthwise and leave the thinner ends whole. Slice the parsnips and the carrots crosswise on an angle into 2-inch lengths.

3. In a 9 x 13-inch baking pan, toss the parsnips and carrots with the oil and salt. Roast, tossing occasionally, for 30 minutes, or until the vegetables are tender and golden brown.

4. Sprinkle with the lemon juice and serve.

Per serving: 128 calories • 2g protein • 5g fat (0.5g saturated) • 6g fiber • 21g carbohydrate • 408mg sodium • 32mg magnesium

Cooking for One: In a small baking pan, toss a total of ⅓ pound parsnips and carrots (prepared as directed) with 1 teaspoon oil and a scant ¼ teaspoon coarse salt. Roast, tossing occasionally, for 20 to 25 minutes, or until tender and lightly browned. Sprinkle with a scant teaspoon of lemon juice.

Rutabaga Mash

Hands-On Time: 10 minutes | **Total Time:** 25 minutes | **Makes:** 4 (1-cup) servings

Rutabaga—also called orange turnip or swede—is milder than a white turnip and has a slight smoky sweetness to it. It matches beautifully with the spiciness of ginger and the richness of coconut milk. Serve the mash alongside grilled pork or turkey.

2 pounds rutabaga, peeled and cut into 1-inch chunks

1 piece (about 1 inch) fresh ginger, peeled and grated or finely minced

1½ teaspoons salt

½ cup light coconut milk

BELLY BUDDIES:
Rutabaga, ginger, coconut milk

1. In a large saucepan of boiling water, cook the rutabaga, ginger, and 1 teaspoon of the salt for 10 to 15 minutes, or until the rutabaga is very tender.

2. Drain and return to the pot. With a potato masher, mash the rutabaga with the coconut milk and the remaining ½ teaspoon salt. Serve hot.

Per serving: 104 calories • 3g protein • 2.5g fat (2g saturated) • 5g fiber • 20g carbohydrate • 381mg sodium • 46mg magnesium

Cooking for One: Cook ½ pound rutabaga chunks in a small saucepan of boiling water with 1 teaspoon grated fresh ginger and ½ teaspoon salt. Drain and mash with 2 tablespoons coconut milk and ⅛ teaspoon salt.

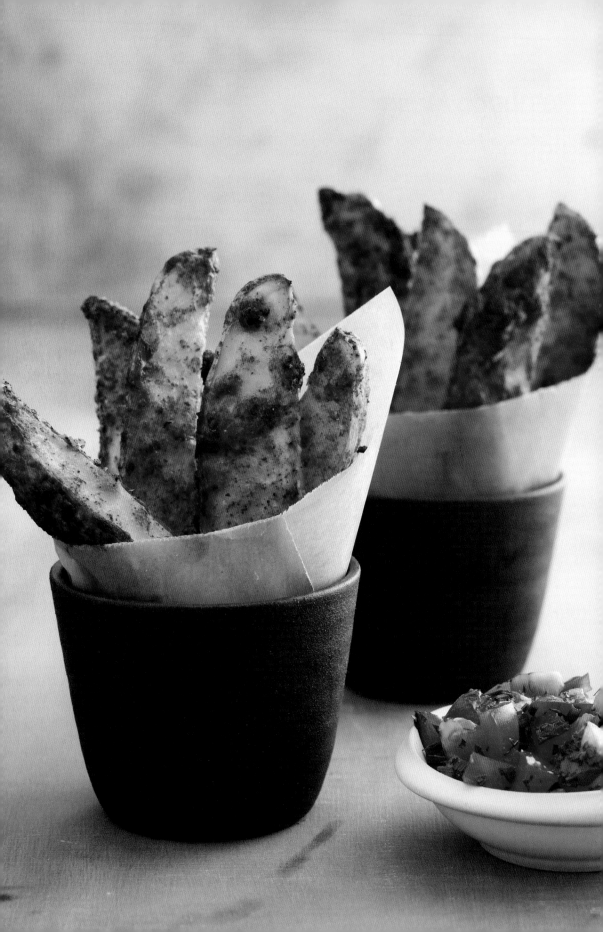

Parmesan Steak Fries

Hands-On Time: 20 minutes | **Total Time:** 1 hour | **Makes:** 4 (4-fries) servings

Ancho chile powder gives a little kick to the crisp fries. We've left the skin on the potatoes for added fiber, but feel free to remove it, if you prefer. Serve these with Barbecue-Glazed Flank Steak (page 129). Top them with the tomato relish from Chicken-Fried Pork with Fresh Tomato Relish (page 135) to avoid the need for ketchup, which often contains carb-dense FODMAP-full sugar.

Olive oil cooking spray

2 russet (baking) potatoes (1 pound total), scrubbed

2 large egg whites

1 tablespoon water

½ cup grated Parmesan cheese

¾ teaspoon ancho chile powder or chipotle chile powder

½ teaspoon coarse (kosher) salt

BELLY BUDDIES: Olive oil, potatoes, eggs

1. Preheat the oven to 450°F. Line a baking sheet with foil or parchment paper, and coat it with cooking spray.

2. Cut each potato lengthwise into 8 wedges. In a large bowl, whisk together the egg whites and water. Place the cheese in a shallow bowl and stir in the chile powder.

3. Add the potatoes to the bowl of egg whites and toss to coat. Lift the potatoes out of the bowl, letting the excess drip off. Dip the skinless sides of the potatoes in the cheese mixture and transfer them to the baking sheet, setting them skin side down.

4. Bake for 35 to 40 minutes, or until the potatoes are browned in spots and firm-tender. Sprinkle with the salt and serve hot.

Per serving: 150 calories • 8g protein • 4g fat (2g saturated) • 1.5g fiber • 21g carbohydrate • 434mg sodium • 33mg magnesium

Cooking for One: Cut 1 small baking potato (about 4 ounces) into 4 lengthwise wedges. Dip each wedge into 1 egg white beaten with 1 teaspoon water. Coat the wedges with 2 tablespoons Parmesan combined with ¼ teaspoon ancho chile powder. Bake as directed. Sprinkle with ⅛ teaspoon coarse salt.

Home Fries

Hands-On Time: 15 minutes | **Total Time:** 50 minutes | **Makes:** 4 (1¼-cup) servings

Who doesn't love the home fries you get at a diner or coffee shop? Here buttery Yukon Gold potatoes get oven-fried along with bell pepper and scallions, for great taste and a modest number of calories.

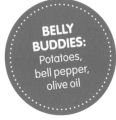

BELLY BUDDIES: Potatoes, bell pepper, olive oil

1¼ pounds Yukon Gold potatoes, well scrubbed and cut into 1-inch chunks

1 yellow bell pepper, diced

½ cup sliced scallion greens or snipped chives

1 tablespoon plus 2 teaspoons extra-virgin olive oil

½ teaspoon coarse (kosher) salt

1. Preheat the oven to 375°F.

2. In a large bowl, toss together the potatoes, bell pepper, scallions, oil, and salt.

3. Transfer to a small rimmed baking sheet and cover with foil. Bake for 20 minutes, or until the potatoes have started to soften. Uncover and continue cooking, tossing once or twice, for 10 to 12 minutes, or until the potatoes are browned and tender.

Per serving: 173 calories • 4g protein • 6g fat (1g saturated) • 3.5g fiber • 28g carbohydrate • 250mg sodium • 41mg magnesium

Cooking for One: Toss 5 ounces potatoes with ¼ diced yellow pepper, 2 tablespoons scallions, 1¼ teaspoons oil, and ⅛ teaspoon salt. Place on a small baking sheet, cover with foil, and bake as directed.

Brown Rice Pilaf with Melted Carrots

Hands-On Time: 15 minutes | **Total Time:** 35 minutes | **Makes:** 4 servings

Shredding the carrots, rather than slicing or dicing them, enables them to get meltingly tender as they cook. For the sweetest carrots, look for those that are of the same thickness from top to bottom. Resist the temptation to buy carrots with their greens attached—they are no fresher or sweeter than others, but are usually more expensive. If you can't find carrot juice, increase the carrots to 2 and increase the water to 1 cup.

2 teaspoons Roasted Garlic Oil (page 54) or extra-virgin olive oil

1 large carrot, shredded

½ cup quick-cooking brown rice

½ cup carrot juice

½ cup water

2 plum tomatoes, coarsely chopped

½ teaspoon salt

¼ teaspoon black pepper

2 tablespoons coarsely chopped pecans

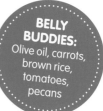

BELLY BUDDIES: Olive oil, carrots, brown rice, tomatoes, pecans

1. In a medium saucepan, heat the oil over medium heat. Add the carrot and cook, stirring frequently, for 3 minutes, or until tender.

2. Add the rice, carrot juice, water, tomatoes, salt, and pepper and bring to a boil. Reduce to a simmer, cover, and cook for 17 to 20 minutes, or until the rice is tender and the liquid has been absorbed.

3. Stir in the pecans and serve.

Per serving: 155 calories • 3g protein • 5.5g fat (0.5g saturated) • 3g fiber • 24g carbohydrate • 328mg sodium • 47mg magnesium

Cooking for One: Sauté 1 small shredded carrot in ½ teaspoon oil until tender. Add 2 tablespoons each quick-cooking brown rice, carrot juice, and water. Stir in ½ plum tomato (chopped), ⅛ teaspoon salt, and a pinch of pepper. Cover and simmer until tender. Stir in 1½ teaspoons chopped pecans.

Herbed Tricolor Quinoa

Hands-On Time: 20 minutes | **Total Time:** 40 minutes plus soaking time | **Makes:** 4 (¾-cup) servings

Quinoa comes in a variety of colors—white, red, and black. You can buy packages of tricolor quinoa, or buy them individually and make your own mix. This recipe also works for just one color of quinoa. Quinoa is gluten-free, low-FODMAP, carb-light, and fiber-rich, making it a top grain for healthy digestion—plus it tastes great!

BELLY BUDDIES:
Quinoa, olive oil, carrot

⅔ cup tricolor quinoa

4 teaspoons extra-virgin olive oil

1 carrot, halved lengthwise and thinly sliced crosswise

1 small fennel bulb, stalks discarded, bulb halved lengthwise and thinly sliced crosswise

½ teaspoon crumbled dried rosemary

½ teaspoon salt

⅛ teaspoon black pepper

1⅓ cups water

½ cup fresh parsley, coarsely chopped

2 tablespoons snipped chives

1. Place the quinoa in a fine-mesh sieve and rinse with cold water; drain well.

2. Meanwhile, in a medium saucepan, heat 2 teaspoons of the oil over medium-low heat. Add the carrot and fennel and cook, stirring frequently, for 5 minutes, or until the vegetables are crisp-tender.

3. Add the drained quinoa, rosemary, salt, and pepper and stir to combine. Add the 1⅓ cups water and bring to a boil. Reduce to a simmer, cover, and cook for 17 minutes, or until the quinoa is tender and the liquid has been absorbed.

4. Stir in the parsley, chives, and the remaining 2 teaspoons oil and serve hot.

Per serving: 172 calories • 5g protein • 6.5g fat (1g saturated) • 4.5g fiber • 25g carbohydrate • 337mg sodium • 72mg magnesium

Cooking for One: Make the whole batch and refrigerate the leftovers in ¾-cup portions. Serve at room temperature or chilled.

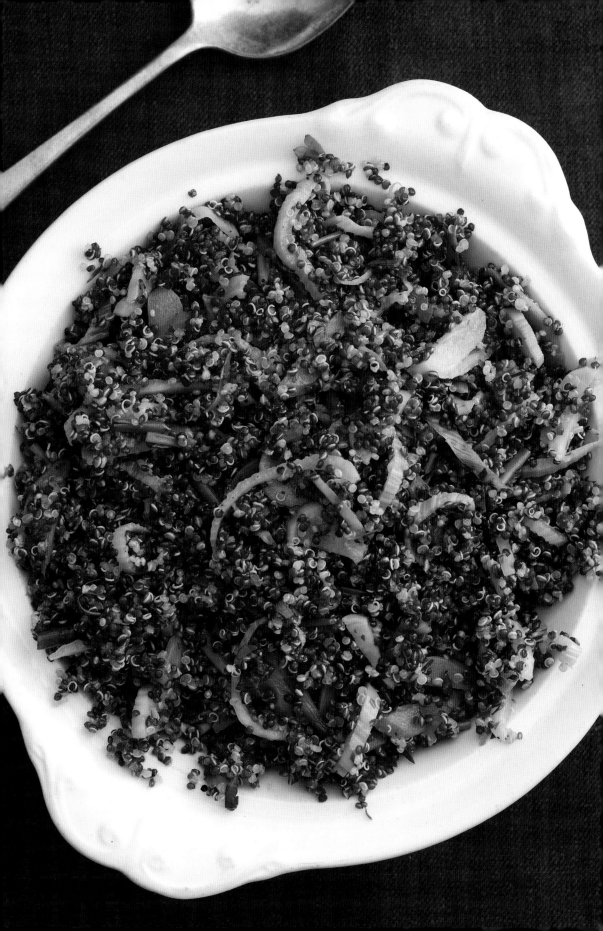

Sunny Kasha

Hands-On Time: 5 minutes | **Total Time:** 15 minutes | **Makes:** 4 (⅔-cup) servings

Do not try to make this with coarse, medium, or fine-grain kasha, or you'll end up with mush. Serve the kasha alongside Lemon Chicken Under a Brick (page 139) and a steamed vegetable, such as green beans or carrots.

BELLY BUDDIES: Buckwheat, tomatoes, sunflower seeds, olive oil, summer squash

- 4 cups water
- ½ cup whole-grain kasha (roasted buckwheat groats)
- ¼ cup finely diced dry-pack sun-dried tomatoes
- 1 teaspoon salt
- 2 tablespoons hulled sunflower seeds
- 1 teaspoon Roasted Garlic Oil (page 54) or extra-virgin olive oil
- 1 small yellow summer squash, finely diced

1. In a medium saucepan, bring the water to a boil. Add the kasha, sun-dried tomatoes, and salt and cook for 6 to 8 minutes, or until tender but not mushy. Drain and return to the saucepan.

2. Meanwhile, in a small skillet, combine the sunflower seeds and oil and cook, stirring, over medium-high heat for 1 to 2 minutes, or until the seeds start to take on color. Add to the cooked kasha and toss to combine.

Per serving: 122 calories • 4g protein • 4g fat (0.5g saturated) • 3.5g fiber • 20g carbohydrate • 70mg sodium • 73mg magnesium

Oat Risotto

Hands-On Time: 10 minutes | **Total Time:** 30 minutes | **Makes:** 4 (½-cup) servings

In Italy, a risotto would be served as a first course, all by itself, but in this country we are more inclined to have it as a side dish. Serve the risotto as a bed for a simple piece of grilled meat or chicken. Unlike a rice-based risotto, this dish gets its creaminess not just from starch but also from the oats' heart-healthy soluble fiber.

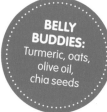

BELLY BUDDIES: Turmeric, oats, olive oil, chia seeds

3 cups low-sodium chicken broth (look for brands with no onions or garlic)

½ cup water

½ teaspoon turmeric

¼ teaspoon salt

⅔ cup steel-cut oats

1 teaspoon extra-virgin olive oil

2 teaspoons chia seeds

¼ cup grated Parmesan cheese

1. In a nonstick medium saucepan, combine the broth, water, turmeric, and salt and bring to a boil over high heat. Stir in the oats, reduce to a simmer, cover, and cook for 15 minutes. Set a sieve over a small saucepan and drain the oats. Set the oats aside and place the small saucepan of broth over a low flame to keep warm.

2. Wipe out the first saucepan and place over medium heat. Add the oil and chia seeds and cook for 45 seconds, or until fragrant.

3. Add the partially cooked oats and ½ cup of the warm broth to the saucepan with the chia seeds. Cook the oats over medium-low heat, stirring, until the liquid is absorbed. Continue adding the warm broth in ½-cup amounts and cook, stirring constantly, for 8 to 10 minutes, or until the oats are firm-tender and the mixture is creamy but not soupy (like porridge).

4. Stir in the cheese and serve hot.

Per serving: 153 calories • 7g protein • 5g fat (1.5g saturated) • 3.5g fiber • 20g carbohydrate • 274mg sodium • 8mg magnesium

If you have gluten issues: Choose gluten-free brands of chicken broth, oats, and chia seeds.

Cooking for One: Reduce the chicken broth to ¾ cup and the water to 2 tablespoons. Season with ⅛ teaspoon turmeric and a pinch of salt. Reduce the oats to a scant 3 tablespoons and cook as directed, but in a small saucepan. Sauté ½ teaspoon chia seeds in ¼ teaspoon oil. Add the oats and cook, adding the broth as directed, but in about three additions. Stir in 1 tablespoon Parmesan at the end.

Upside-Down Pineapple Corn Skillet Cake

Also makes a nice breakfast

Chapter 10

Desserts

INDULGE WITH SWEET STOMACH SOOTHERS

Cantaloupe Granita

Hands-On Time: 10 minutes | **Total Time:** 10 minutes plus freezing time | **Makes:** 4 (1-cup) servings

A granita is a type of frozen fruit dessert that is similar to a sorbet, but it's granular rather than smooth textured. Once you've frozen the melon (try to get a super ripe one for the most flavor), the dessert takes only minutes to prepare. One cup of cantaloupe exceeds your vitamin A and C needs for the day—a tasty way to keep your immune and digestive systems strong!

BELLY BUDDIES: Cantaloupe, lemon

4 cups small chunks cantaloupe (about 1¼ pounds)

2 tablespoons fresh lemon juice

1. Spread the cantaloupe out in a baking pan or on a baking sheet and freeze for 2 hours, or until almost solid.

2. Transfer the frozen melon to a food processor along with the lemon juice and pulse until the consistency of a granita. Serve immediately.

Per serving: 55 calories • 1g protein • 0.5g fat (0g saturated) • 1.5g fiber • 13g carbohydrate • 25mg sodium • 19mg magnesium

Cooking for One: Freeze 1 cup cantaloupe cubes, then pulse in a food processor with 1½ teaspoons lemon juice.

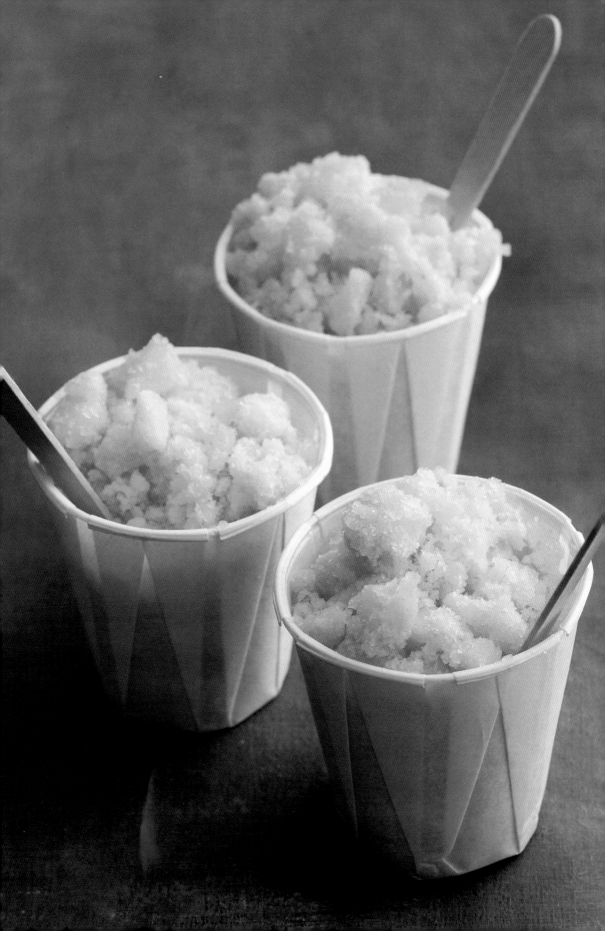

Raspberry Fool

Hands-On Time: 20 minutes | **Total Time:** 20 minutes plus freezing time | **Makes:** 4 (2-slice) servings

A "fool" is a super simple dessert made with sweetened berry puree and whipped cream folded together. We took the idea and turned it into a frozen dessert, subbing in Greek yogurt for whipped cream and adding a little banana for a smooth texture and some natural sweetness. You could easily swap in frozen mixed berries or strawberries for the raspberries, but we love the fiber boost in raspberries: 1 cup provides 8 grams of belly-friendly fiber!

BELLY BUDDIES: Raspberries, banana, maple syrup, Greek yogurt

12 ounces frozen unsweetened raspberries, thawed

1 banana (5 ounces)

3 tablespoons pure maple syrup

½ teaspoon ground cardamom

⅔ cup nonfat plain Greek yogurt

1. In a food processor, puree the raspberries. Set a fine-mesh sieve over a large bowl and strain the puree through the sieve. Discard the seeds.

2. Place the banana, maple syrup, and cardamom in the food processor (no need to clean it first) and puree. Fold the banana puree into the raspberry puree. Fold in the yogurt.

3. Line an 8 x 4-inch loaf pan with plastic wrap, leaving an overhang all around. Spoon the mixture into the loaf pan and fold the overhang over to cover the top. Freeze for at least 4 hours or up to several days.

4. To serve, open the plastic wrap and invert the loaf onto a serving platter. Remove the wrap and cut the loaf into 8 slices, serving 2 slices per person.

Per serving: 128 calories • 4g protein • 0g fat (0g saturated) • 4.5g fiber • 30g carbohydrate • 16mg sodium • 13mg magnesium

If you have gluten issues: Choose a gluten-free brand of Greek yogurt.

Blueberry-Lime Cream Parfait

Hands-On Time: 15 minutes | **Total Time:** 15 minutes | **Makes:** 4 servings

This parfait tastes like a cheesecake but without the crust—or the calories. Blueberries are one of the top belly-friendly super foods: Rich in polyphenols, which are key inflammation busters, a full cup has only 84 calories and 3½ grams of filling fiber.

BELLY BUDDIES: Greek yogurt, blueberries, lime

- 3 ounces ⅓-less-fat cream cheese, at room temperature (6 tablespoons)
- 2 tablespoons plus 2 teaspoons light brown sugar
- 1 cup nonfat plain Greek yogurt
- 3 cups blueberries
- 1 teaspoon grated lime zest
- 1 tablespoon fresh lime juice

1. In a medium bowl, combine the cream cheese and 2 tablespoons of the brown sugar and mash together with a spoon. Add the yogurt, stirring until well combined.

2. In a separate bowl, toss the blueberries with the lime zest, lime juice, and the remaining 2 teaspoons brown sugar. Lightly mash some of the berries with a potato masher or a fork, leaving most of the berries whole.

3. Layer the cream cheese mixture and the berries (and their juices) into 4 wine glasses, ending with a dollop of the cream cheese mixture. Serve immediately or chill until ready to serve.

Per serving: 183 calories • 8g protein • 5g fat (2.5g saturated) • 2.5g fiber • 29g carbohydrate • 96mg sodium • 10mg magnesium

If you have gluten issues: Choose a gluten-free brand of Greek yogurt.

Cooking for One: Mash 1½ tablespoons cream cheese with 1½ teaspoons brown sugar. Stir in ¼ cup Greek yogurt. Lightly mash ¾ cup blueberries with ½ teaspoon brown sugar, ¼ teaspoon grated lime zest, and ¾ teaspoon lime juice. Layer into a parfait glass.

Strawberry Mousse

Hands-On Time: 10 minutes | **Total Time:** 10 minutes plus chilling time | **Makes:** 4 servings

Try the mousse with different belly-friendly fruits, such as blueberries, raspberries, or bananas. You'll need about 1 cup of fruit.

BELLY BUDDIES:
Strawberries, maple syrup, Greek yogurt

½ pound strawberries, hulled and halved

1 envelope (¼ ounce) unflavored gelatin

¼ cup water

¼ cup plus 2 tablespoons pure maple syrup

½ teaspoon vanilla extract

1 cup nonfat plain Greek yogurt

1. In a food processor, process the berries to a smooth puree. (Leave the puree in the processor.)

2. In a small bowl, sprinkle the gelatin over the water. Let sit for 2 to 3 minutes to soften.

3. In a small saucepan, heat the maple syrup over medium-low heat for 1 minute, or until it begins to boil. Remove from the heat. Scrape the softened gelatin mixture into the hot maple syrup and stir well to dissolve the gelatin.

4. Add the gelatin-maple mixture to the strawberry puree and process to blend well.

5. In a medium bowl, whisk the vanilla into the yogurt. Keep whisking the yogurt to lighten it, then whisk in the strawberry puree. Spoon into four 6- to 8-ounce ramekins or goblets, or a 4-cup serving bowl and chill for 3 to 4 hours, or until set (the shorter time for the individual servings).

Per serving: 134 calories • 7g protein • 0g fat (0g saturated) • 1g fiber • 27g carbohydrate • 29mg sodium • 14mg magnesium

If you have gluten issues: Choose a gluten-free brand of Greek yogurt.

Toasted Coconut Panna Cotta

Hands-On Time: 15 minutes | **Total Time:** 15 minutes plus chilling time |
Makes: 8 servings

In Italian, *panna cotta* means "cooked cream." Here we've used light coconut milk to make this creamy gelatin dessert, thus avoiding the belly-bulging calories and tummy-troubling lactose of cream.

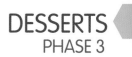

BELLY BUDDIES: Coconut milk, coconut

- 1 envelope (¼ ounce) unflavored gelatin
- 2⅔ cups light coconut milk
- ⅓ cup packed turbinado or light brown sugar
- ⅛ teaspoon salt
- 2 tablespoons unsweetened shredded coconut

1. In a small saucepan, sprinkle the gelatin over 1⅔ cups of the coconut milk and let stand for 5 minutes, or until the gelatin is softened.

2. Place the saucepan over low heat and stir in the sugar and salt and cook for 2 minutes, or until the gelatin has dissolved. Stir in the remaining 1 cup coconut milk.

3. Divide the mixture among eight 6-ounce ramekins or custard cups and chill for 2 hours, or until set.

4. Meanwhile, place the coconut in a small skillet and cook over low heat, stirring constantly, for 3 minutes, or until toasted and golden brown. Remove from the pan to stop the cooking.

5. To serve, sprinkle 1½ teaspoons of the coconut over each panna cotta.

Per serving: 100 calories • 1g protein • 5g fat (4g saturated) • 1g fiber • 14g carbohydrate • 64mg sodium • 0mg magnesium

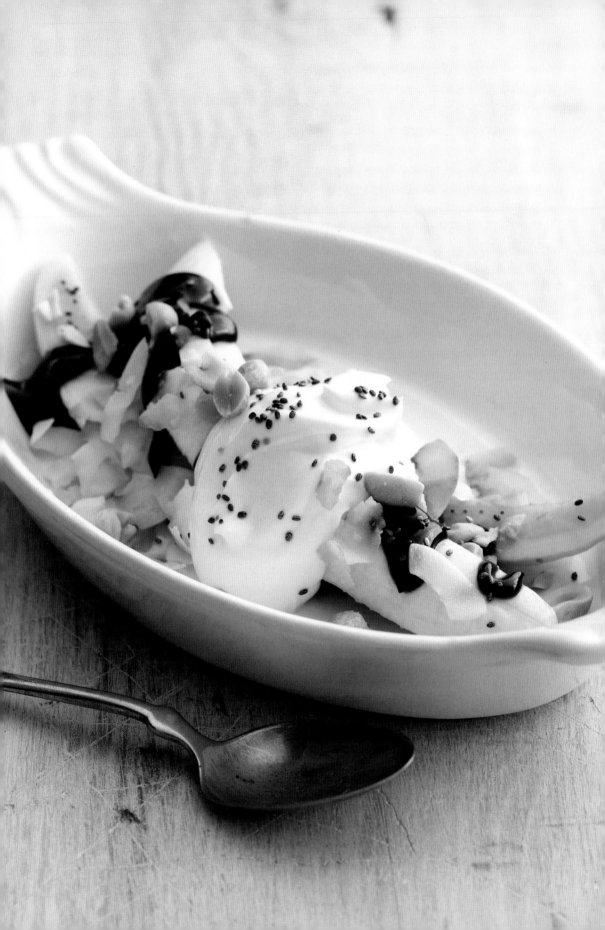

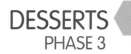

"Banana Splits"

Hands-On Time: 15 minutes | **Total Time:** 15 minutes | **Makes:** 4 servings

Greek yogurt sweetened with belly-friendly maple syrup stands in for the traditional ice cream topping in this classic dessert. We've used peanuts for the crushed nuts that often top the banana, and toasted coconut and chia seeds for added crunch and a dash of tummy-taming fiber and easy to digest anti-inflammation fats.

1 ounce semisweet chocolate, coarsely chopped

2 tablespoons unsweetened shredded coconut

½ cup nonfat plain Greek yogurt

2 tablespoons pure maple syrup

2 bananas (6 ounces each), peeled, halved crosswise and lengthwise

2 tablespoons coarsely chopped unsalted peanuts

1 teaspoon chia seeds

BELLY BUDDIES: Dark chocolate, Greek yogurt, maple syrup, bananas, peanuts, chia seeds

1. In a small bowl, set over (not in) a pan of simmering water, melt the chocolate.

2. In a small, dry skillet, toast the coconut over low heat, stirring constantly, for 3 minutes, or until golden brown.

3. In a small bowl, stir together the yogurt and maple syrup.

4. Divide the bananas among 4 shallow dessert bowls. Drizzle with the melted chocolate, spoon the yogurt mixture on top. Sprinkle with the coconut, peanuts, and chia seeds.

Per serving: 203 calories • 5g protein • 7g fat (3.5g saturated) • 4g fiber • 33g carbohydrate • 14mg sodium • 36mg magnesium

If you have gluten issues: Choose gluten-free brands of Greek yogurt and chia seeds.

Cooking for One: Melt ¼ ounce chocolate and toast 1½ teaspoons coconut. Blend 2 tablespoons yogurt with 1½ teaspoons maple syrup. Top ½ banana with the chocolate, yogurt mixture, toasted coconut, 1½ teaspoons chopped peanuts, and ¼ teaspoon chia seeds.

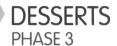

Berry-Studded Rice Pudding

Hands-On Time: 10 minutes | **Total Time:** 25 minutes plus cooling time | **Makes:** 4 (1-cup) servings

Quick-cooking brown rice has all the nutrients of regular brown rice but cooks in a fraction of the time. Look for it on the grocery shelf next to regular rice, but take care not to buy the "minute" rice, as its texture is not as firm.

BELLY BUDDIES: Brown rice, blueberries, strawberries

⅓ cup water

⅛ teaspoon salt

1¼ cups unsweetened rice milk

⅔ cup quick-cooking brown rice

2 tablespoons light brown sugar

1 cup blueberries

1 cup sliced strawberries or raspberries

1. In a small saucepan, combine the water, salt, and 1 cup of the rice milk and bring to a boil over high heat. Add the rice, reduce to a simmer, cover, and cook for 12 to 15 minutes, or until the rice is tender.

2. Remove from the heat and stir in the brown sugar and the remaining ¼ cup rice milk. Cool to room temperature, then stir in the blueberries and strawberries. Serve at room temperature or chilled.

Per serving: 149 calories • 2g protein • 1.5g fat (0g saturated) • 4g fiber • 34g carbohydrate • 106mg sodium • 18mg magnesium

Cooking for One: In a small saucepan, bring ¼ cup rice milk, 1½ tablespoons water, and a pinch of salt to a boil. Add 1½ tablespoons quick-cooking brown rice and cook until tender. Stir in 1 tablespoon rice milk and 1½ teaspoons brown sugar. Cool to room temperature and stir in ¼ cup each blueberries and strawberries.

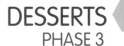
Three-Citrus Coconut Macaroons

Hands-On Time: 10 minutes | **Total Time:** 35 minutes | **Makes:** 18 macaroons

The grated zest from three citrus fruits peaks the flavor of these cookies. The next time you juice any citrus, pop the shell into the freezer. Then when you need zest, simply grate the frozen shell. Citrus fruits are low in FODMAPs and rich in immune-boosting, fat-releasing vitamin C.

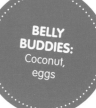

BELLY BUDDIES: Coconut, eggs

4 ounces unsweetened shredded coconut

¼ cup packed turbinado sugar

½ teaspoon grated lemon zest

½ teaspoon grated lime zest

½ teaspoon grated orange zest

⅛ teaspoon salt

3 large egg whites

1. Preheat the oven to 325°F. Line a baking sheet with parchment paper.

2. In a food processor, combine the coconut, sugar, lemon zest, lime zest, orange zest, and salt. Add the egg whites and pulse until well combined.

3. Shape the mixture into 18 rounds. Place on the baking sheet and bake for 20 to 25 minutes, or until lightly colored and set.

4. Transfer to a wire rack to cool completely. Store on the countertop in an airtight container for up to 1 week.

Per macaroon: 66 calories • 1g protein • 4.5g fat (4g saturated) • 1g fiber • 5g carbohydrate • 28mg sodium • 1mg magnesium

Almond Biscotti

Hands-On Time: 15 minutes | **Total Time:** 1 hour 20 minutes | **Makes:** 20 cookies

Typically biscotti are baked in a free-form loaf, which, when you cut it into cookies, always leaves uneven, slightly rounded "heels" that get wasted. This method uses a loaf pan, yielding perfectly shaped biscotti. Using almond flour and cornmeal instead of regular flour reduces the carb density of these crunchy treats. But because they are still a little more carb-dense than most of the foods on the 21-Day Tummy plan, be sure to stick with Phase 1 recipes and other naturally carb-light foods for the rest of your meal.

BELLY BUDDIES:
Maple syrup, egg

Olive oil cooking spray
4 tablespoons cornmeal
1¼ cups almond flour
¼ cup cornstarch
1 teaspoon ground cardamom
¾ teaspoon ground cinnamon
¼ teaspoon baking powder
¼ teaspoon salt
⅓ cup pure maple syrup
1 large egg

1. Preheat the oven to 350°F. Coat an 8 x 4-inch loaf pan with cooking spray. Dust with 1 tablespoon of the cornmeal.

2. In a large bowl, stir together the almond flour, cornstarch, cardamom, cinnamon, baking powder, salt, and the remaining 3 tablespoons cornmeal. Make a well in the center and stir in the maple syrup and egg until incorporated.

3. Transfer the dough to the loaf pan and press into the bottom of the pan, smoothing the top of the dough. Cover with foil and bake for 50 minutes, or until set.

4. Run a metal spatula around the edge of the pan and invert the loaf onto a wire rack to cool slightly. Reduce the oven temperature to 325°F.

5. With a serrated knife, cut the loaf crosswise into twenty ½-inch slices. Arrange them on a baking sheet and bake for 15 minutes, or until the slices are dry. Cool on a wire rack.

Per cookie: 73 calories • 2g protein • 4g fat (0.5g saturated) • 1g fiber • 8g carbohydrate • 43mg sodium • 22mg magnesium

If you have gluten issues: Choose a gluten-free brand of baking powder.

Chocolate-Chip Walnut Cookies

Hands-On Time: 25 minutes | **Total Time:** 1 hour 5 minutes | **Makes:** 36 cookies

These cookies bake up crisp, but if you'd prefer them a little chewy, bake them for 3 minutes less than the given time. If you've got 2 large baking sheets, you can bake both batches at the same time, switching the sheets from top to bottom midway through, which would reduce the total time by about 20 minutes. Store for up to 2 days in an airtight container, or, wrap and freeze up to 3 months; these can be eaten straight out of the freezer, or thawed at room temperature. Because these cookies are a little more carb-dense than most of the foods on the 21-Day Tummy plan, be sure to stick with Phase 1 recipes and other naturally carb-light foods for the rest of your meal.

1 cup brown rice flour
½ cup cornstarch
½ teaspoon baking soda
½ teaspoon salt
⅓ cup extra-virgin olive oil
¾ cup packed light brown sugar

2 large egg whites
1 teaspoon vanilla extract
½ cup semisweet mini chocolate chips
⅓ cup chopped walnuts

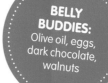

BELLY BUDDIES:
Olive oil, eggs, dark chocolate, walnuts

1. Preheat the oven to 350°F. Line a large baking sheet with parchment paper.

2. In a medium bowl, stir together the flour, cornstarch, baking soda, and salt.

3. In a large bowl, with an electric mixer, beat together the oil and brown sugar until well combined. One at a time, add the egg whites, beating well after each addition. Beat in the vanilla.

4. With the mixer on low speed, beat in the flour mixture until well combined. Mix in the chocolate chips and walnuts.

5. Drop the dough by rounded teaspoons onto the baking sheet, spacing them 2 inches apart. Bake for 17 minutes, or until set. Cool for 1 minute on the baking sheet, then transfer to a wire rack to cool completely.

Per cookie: 89 calories • 1g protein • 4.5g fat (1g saturated) • 0.5g fiber • 12g carbohydrate • 55mg sodium • 4mg magnesium

Chocolate-Covered Peanut Butter Cookies

Hands-On Time: 10 minutes | **Total Time:** 25 minutes plus cooling | **Makes:** 2 dozen cookies

These moist cookies have not a speck of flour in them, yet they rise just like little cakes. You need 4 chocolate chips for the top of each cookie, which is approximately ¼ cup of chips. The cookies freeze well, so spread them on a baking sheet to freeze, then transfer to a freezer container. They will keep well for 1 month. Let thaw at room temperature to eat (do not thaw in the microwave).

BELLY BUDDIES:
Peanut butter, banana, eggs, dark chocolate

1 cup natural peanut butter

1 banana (7 ounces), cut into small chunks

¼ cup packed turbinado sugar or light brown sugar

1 large egg

2 large egg whites

¼ cup semisweet chocolate chips

1. Preheat the oven to 350°F. Line a large baking sheet with parchment paper or a nonstick liner. If your baking sheet is not large enough to accommodate 2 dozen 2-inch cookies, bake in batches.

2. In a bowl, with an electric mixer, beat together the peanut butter, banana, sugar, whole egg, and egg whites until smooth. Spoon the batter by tablespoon about 1 inch apart onto the baking sheet.

3. Bake for 14 to 16 minutes, or until puffed and browned around the edges.

4. Remove from the oven, but leave the cookies on the pan for 5 minutes. While they're still hot, place 4 chocolate chips on top of each.

5. Transfer the cookies to a wire rack to cool. As soon as the chips are melted, spread them over the top of the cookie. Let sit until the chocolate sets.

Per cookie: 96 calories • 3g protein • 6g fat (1g saturated) • 1g fiber • 8g carbohydrate • 8mg sodium • 1mg magnesium

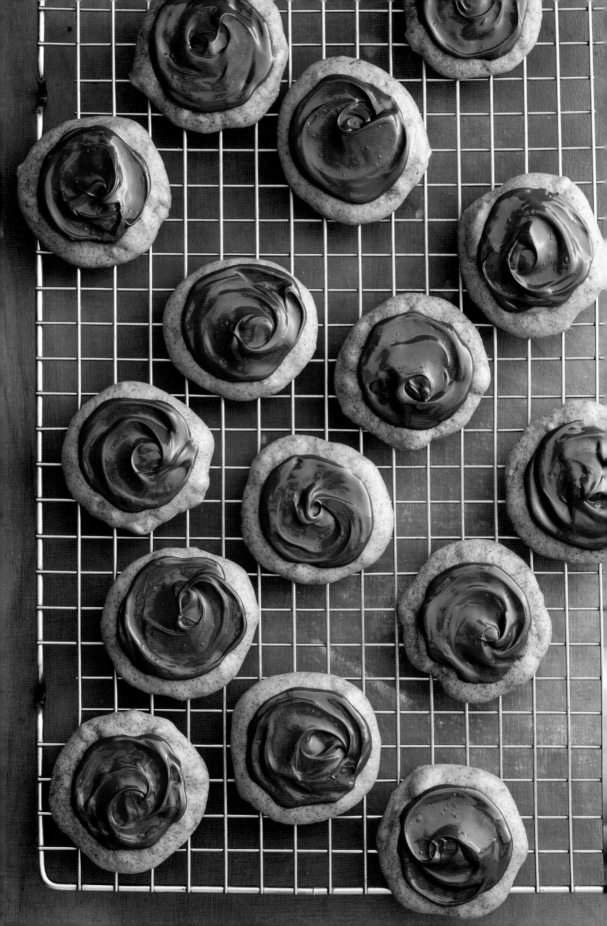

Creamy Orange-Lemon Bars

Hands-On Time: 15 minutes | **Total Time:** 55 minutes plus cooling time |
Makes: 12 bars

These dessert bars freeze extremely well, so before you're tempted to eat more than one, spread them out on a baking sheet and freeze solid. Then transfer to a freezer container. Let them thaw at room temperature to eat, or give them a 20- to 30-second zap in the microwave.

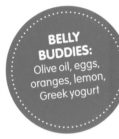

BELLY BUDDIES:
Olive oil, eggs, oranges, lemon, Greek yogurt

You can also get a little creative with this recipe by subbing in other fruit juices. To swap out the orange juice, choose a fruit juice that has about the same balance of sweet to tart. Try unsweetened pineapple juice, raspberry juice, tangerine juice, or white grape juice. (If you happen to have oranges on hand, keep the grated zest in the recipe; otherwise, just omit.) Then for the lemon juice, you can substitute unsweetened cranberry juice or lime juice—or, if your market carries them, the juice of Meyer lemons. (For the zest, use it if you have it, but otherwise just omit.)

And don't forget to play around with the crust. It would be quite nice with some "warm" spices: Try adding a pinch of cinnamon, nutmeg, cardamom, or allspice to the dry ingredients. But don't go overboard; keep the spicing subtle.

Olive oil cooking spray

CRUST

- ⅓ cup brown rice flour
- ¼ cup almond flour
- ¼ cup coconut flour
- 2 tablespoons dark brown sugar
- ¼ teaspoon salt
- 2 tablespoons water
- 2 tablespoons olive oil

FILLING

- 2 large eggs
- 2 large egg whites
- ½ cup packed turbinado sugar or light brown sugar
- 1 teaspoon grated orange zest
- ⅓ cup fresh orange juice
- 1 teaspoon grated lemon zest
- ⅓ cup fresh lemon juice (about 2 lemons)
- ⅓ cup nonfat plain Greek yogurt
- 2 tablespoons brown rice flour
- ¼ teaspoon salt

1. Preheat the oven to 350°F. Coat an 8 x 8-inch baking pan with cooking spray.

2. **Make the crust:** In a bowl, stir together the rice flour, almond flour, coconut flour, brown sugar, and salt. Add the water and oil and stir with a fork until well distributed. Then use your fingers to rub the liquids into the dry ingredients to make a crumbly dough that will stick together when pinched.

3. Press the dough firmly into the bottom of the baking pan. Bake for 10 to 12 minutes, or until set and lightly browned. Remove from the oven and let cool for 5 minutes. Leave the oven on.

4. **Meanwhile, make the filling:** In a medium bowl, whisk together the whole eggs, egg whites, sugar, orange zest, orange juice, lemon zest, and lemon juice.

5. In a small bowl, beat together the yogurt, flour, and salt. Beat a little of the orange-lemon mixture into the yogurt mixture to loosen it, then whisk all the yogurt mixture back into the orange-lemon mixture until well incorporated.

6. Pour the filling on top of the cooled crust. Bake for 25 to 30 minutes, or until the filling sets and is light golden at the edges. Let cool completely in the pan on a rack before cutting into 12 bars.

Per bar: 133 calories • 4g protein • 4.5g fat (1g saturated) • 1.5g fiber • 20g carbohydrate • 127mg sodium • 10mg magnesium

If you have gluten issues: Choose a gluten-free brand of Greek yogurt.

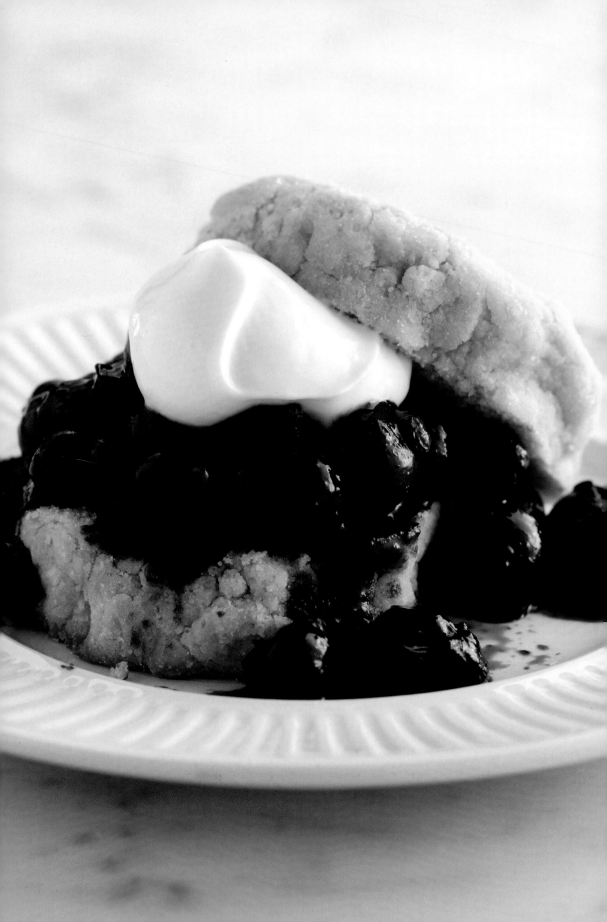

Blueberry Shortcakes

Hands-On Time: 15 minutes | **Total Time:** 30 minutes plus cooling time |
Makes: 6 shortcakes

The shortcakes are sort of like mini scones, so you could bake up a batch of them on their own. Spread them on a baking sheet and freeze solid, then transfer to an airtight freezer container. Thaw at room temperature (not in the microwave). Have one for breakfast with ½ cup nonfat plain Greek yogurt, sweetened with a dash of maple syrup.

SHORTCAKES

- ¾ cup brown rice flour
- ¼ cup almond flour
- 2 teaspoons baking powder
- 2 teaspoons grated lemon zest
- ½ teaspoon salt
- 2 tablespoons coconut oil
- 1 tablespoon pure maple syrup
- 5 tablespoons lactose-free 1% milk

BLUEBERRY COMPOTE

- 1 tablespoon dark brown sugar
- 1 tablespoon water
- 1 teaspoon grated lemon zest
- 1½ cups blueberries

TOPPING

- ¼ cup nonfat plain Greek yogurt
- 2 teaspoons pure maple syrup

BELLY BUDDIES: Maple syrup, blueberries, Greek yogurt

1. Preheat the oven to 400°F. Line a baking sheet with parchment paper.

2. **Make the shortcakes:** In a medium bowl, stir together the rice flour, almond flour, baking powder, lemon zest, and salt. Make a well in the center and add the coconut oil, maple syrup, and milk. Stir together the entire mixture until evenly incorporated.

3. Drop the dough into 6 equal portions on the baking sheet and pat gently to flatten the top, making a biscuit about 2 inches across. Bake for 10 to 12 minutes, or until light brown and risen. Let cool on the pan.

4. **Meanwhile, make the blueberry compote:** In a small saucepan, combine the brown sugar, water, lemon zest, and ¾ cup of the blueberries. Bring to a bubble over medium heat and cook, stirring, for 2 to 3 minutes, or until the berries collapse and turn saucy. Remove from the heat and stir in the remaining ¾ cup whole blueberries.

5. Make the topping: In a small bowl, stir together the yogurt and maple syrup.

(continued on page 282)

(continued from page 281)

Blueberry Shortcakes

6. When ready to serve, carefully split the cakes horizontally, cutting so the bottom is thicker and wider than the top. Spoon about 2 tablespoons berry compote on the bottom, dollop with 2 teaspoons yogurt topping, and replace the top.

Per shortcake: 196 calories • 5g protein • 7.5g fat (4g saturated) • 2g fiber • 30g carbohydrate • 393mg sodium • 18mg magnesium

If you have gluten issues: Choose gluten-free brands of baking powder and Greek yogurt.

Cooking for One: Make the whole batch of shortcakes and freeze the leftover shortcakes, baked but uncut. Refrigerate or freeze the blueberry compote. (Freeze it in ice cube trays; for a single serving, thaw 1 or 2 cubes.) To serve, let a shortcake come to room temperature, then very briefly microwave (10 to 20 seconds) to warm it up before slicing it open. Make the yogurt topping as needed: For each individual serving, lightly sweeten 2 teaspoons yogurt with a generous ¼ teaspoon maple syrup.

Strawberry-Rhubarb Crisp

Hands-On Time: 15 minutes | **Total Time:** 1 hour plus cooling time |
Makes: 6 servings

This classic fruit pie combination also works well as a crisp, in this
case topped with a combination of oats, coconut, and almonds for a
healthful crunch. Rhubarb's tart flavor complements the sweetness of the
strawberries in this recipe. Both fruits are low-FODMAP and fiber-rich and
up your vitamin C intake.

Olive oil cooking spray

TOPPING

½ cup quick-cooking oats

⅓ cup unsweetened shredded
coconut

⅓ cup sliced almonds, coarsely
chopped

Generous pinch of salt

2 tablespoons pure maple
syrup

2 teaspoons extra-virgin olive
oil

FILLING

2 cups thinly sliced rhubarb

1 pound strawberries,
quartered (or cut into eighths
if large)

¼ cup packed light brown sugar

2 tablespoons brown rice flour

¼ teaspoon ground cardamom

Pinch of ground allspice

Pinch of salt

BELLY BUDDIES:
Oats, coconut, maple syrup, olive oil, strawberries

1. Preheat the oven to 375°F. Coat
the sides of an 8 x 8-inch baking
pan with cooking spray.

2. Make the topping: In a small
bowl, toss together the oats,
coconut, almonds, and salt. Add
the maple syrup and oil and stir to
evenly moisten.

3. Make the filling: In a large
bowl, toss together the rhubarb
and strawberries. Sprinkle with
the brown sugar, flour, cardamom,
allspice, and salt and toss well to
coat.

4. Scrape the fruit mixture into
the baking pan. Top evenly with
the oat mixture. Bake for 35 to 45
minutes, or until the top is nicely
browned and the fruit is bubbling.

5. Let stand for 10 minutes
before serving, or serve at room
temperature.

Per serving: 209 calories • 4g protein • 8.5g
fat (3g saturated) • 4.5g fiber • 31g carbohydrate • 54mg sodium • 30mg magnesium

If you have gluten issues: Choose a gluten-
free brand of oats.

Carrot-Pineapple Slices with Cream Cheese Frosting

Hands-On Time: 25 minutes | **Total Time:** 55 minutes plus cooling time |
Makes: 12 slices

Greek yogurt and ⅓-less-fat cream cheese, along with some brown sugar, make for a sweet, yet tangy, topping for this classic treat. We've mixed flours from several carb-light grains (buckwheat, brown rice, oats) for the perfect texture and combination of belly-flattening protein and fiber.

BELLY BUDDIES:
Ginger, olive oil, egg, carrots, pineapple, Greek yogurt

Olive oil cooking spray
¼ cup buckwheat flour
¼ cup brown rice flour
½ cup oat flour
1 teaspoon baking soda
¾ teaspoon ground ginger
½ teaspoon ground cinnamon
¼ teaspoon salt
3 tablespoons olive oil

⅓ cup plus 2 tablespoons packed light brown sugar
1 large egg
1 cup grated carrots
1 can (8 ounces) juice-packed crushed pineapple, drained
¾ cup nonfat plain Greek yogurt
3 ounces ⅓-less-fat cream cheese, at room temperature

1. Preheat the oven to 350°F. Coat an 8 x 8-inch baking pan with cooking spray.

2. In a medium bowl, stir together the flours, baking soda, ginger, cinnamon, and salt.

3. With an electric mixer, beat together the oil and ⅓ cup of the brown sugar. Beat in the egg. Beat in the flour mixture on low speed. Fold in the carrots and pineapple.

4. Scrape the batter into the baking pan and bake for 30 minutes, or until a wooden pick comes out mostly clean.

5. Cool for 10 minutes in the pan, then run a metal spatula around the edge of the cake and invert onto a wire rack to cool.

6. In a medium bowl, beat together the yogurt, cream cheese, and the remaining 2 tablespoons brown sugar until smooth. Spread over the cooled cake.

7. To serve, cut into 12 slices.

Per slice: 144 calories • 3g protein • 6g fat (1.5g saturated) • 1.5g fiber • 20g carbohydrate • 198mg sodium • 13mg magnesium

If you have gluten issues: Choose gluten-free brands of oat flour, Greek yogurt, and buckwheat flour.

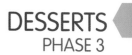

Grape and Almond Custard Cake

Hands-On Time: 10 minutes | **Total Time:** 50 minutes plus cooling time |
Makes: 6 servings

This cake is somewhere between a custard and a cake: moister than cake, firmer than custard. It's based on a home-style French dessert called a clafouti. Store leftovers in the refrigerator.

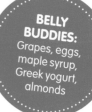

BELLY BUDDIES: Grapes, eggs, maple syrup, Greek yogurt, almonds

Olive oil cooking spray

50 to 60 seedless green grapes (about ¾ pound)

¼ cup plus 2 tablespoons brown rice flour

½ teaspoon baking powder

¼ teaspoon salt

3 large eggs

½ cup lactose-free 1% milk

¼ teaspoon almond extract

3 tablespoons plus 2 teaspoons pure maple syrup

¼ cup plus 2 tablespoons nonfat plain Greek yogurt

2 tablespoons slivered almonds

1. Preheat the oven to 350°F. Coat the bottom and sides of an 8 x 8-inch baking pan with cooking spray. Line the bottom and up two sides of the pan with parchment paper, leaving an overhang. Scatter the grapes over the bottom of the pan to cover it in a single layer.

2. In a bowl, with an electric mixer, beat together the flour, baking powder, and salt. Add the eggs, milk, almond extract, and 3 tablespoons of the maple syrup and beat until well combined. The consistency will be like very loose pancake batter.

3. Pour the batter over the grapes. Bake for 40 minutes, or until golden brown, puffed, and set. Let cool in the pan to lukewarm or room temperature. Lift out of the pan and cut into 6 rectangles.

4. Stir the remaining 2 teaspoons maple syrup into the yogurt. Serve the bars dolloped with the yogurt and sprinkle with the almonds.

Per serving: 183 calories • 7g protein • 5.5g fat (1g saturated) • 1g fiber • 29g carbohydrate • 198mg sodium • 18mg magnesium

If you have gluten issues: Choose gluten-free brands of Greek yogurt and baking powder.

Upside-Down Pineapple Corn Skillet Cake

Hands-On Time: 10 minutes | **Total Time:** 30 minutes plus cooling time | **Makes:** 8 wedges

A wedge of this quick and easy dessert would also make a nice breakfast. It will keep in an airtight container for 2 days in the fridge.

BELLY BUDDIES: Maple syrup, pineapple, Greek yogurt, egg

2 tablespoons coconut oil

6 tablespoons pure maple syrup

7 juice-packed canned pineapple rings

1 cup nonfat plain Greek yogurt

1 cup cornmeal

½ teaspoon salt

½ teaspoon baking powder

¼ teaspoon baking soda

1 large egg

½ cup water

1. Preheat the oven to 375°F. In a 10-inch nonstick skillet, combine the oil and 2 tablespoons of the maple syrup. Add the pineapple rings in a single layer, covering the bottom of the skillet.

2. In a small bowl, stir together ½ cup of the yogurt and 1 tablespoon of the maple syrup. Refrigerate until serving time.

3. In a medium bowl, stir together the cornmeal, salt, baking powder, and baking soda. In a separate bowl, whisk together the egg, water, and the remaining ½ cup yogurt and 3 tablespoons maple syrup.

4. Make a well in the center of the dry ingredients, pour in the egg mixture, and mix together with a spoon. Scrape the batter over the pineapple rings and smooth the top.

5. Bake for 20 minutes, or until set and golden brown. Cool for 5 minutes in the pan, then run a metal spatula around the edge of the pan and invert the cake onto a platter.

6. Cut into 8 wedges and serve with the maple yogurt.

Per wedge: 192 calories • 5g protein • 4.5g fat (3g saturated) • 1g fiber • 34g carbohydrate • 246mg sodium • 10mg magnesium

If you have gluten issues: Choose gluten-free brands of Greek yogurt and baking powder.

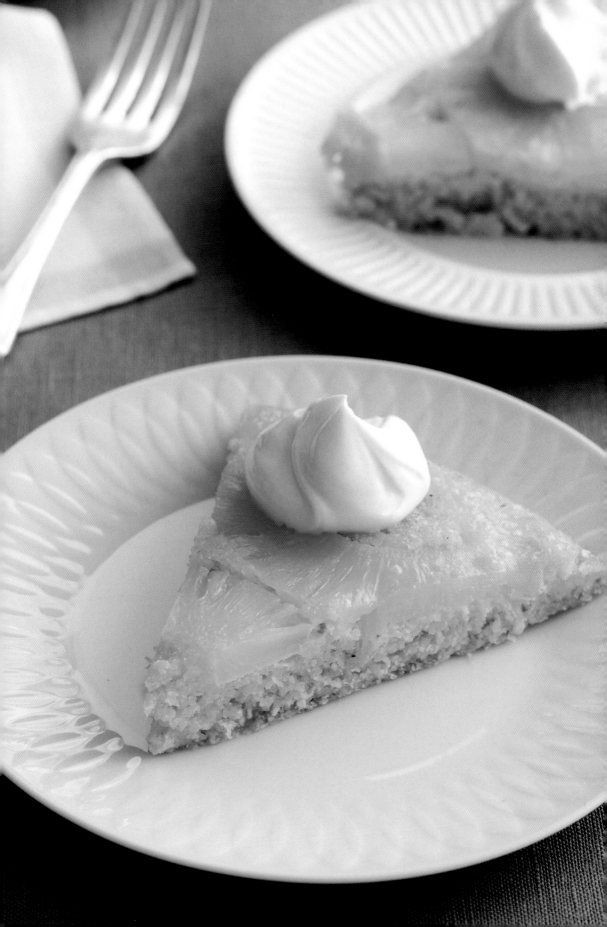

Maple-Glazed Banana Tarts

Hands-On Time: 5 minutes | **Total Time:** 20 minutes | **Makes:** 4 tarts

Corn tortillas are perfect when you need to make a super quick gluten-free tart or pizza. They usually come in pretty big packs, but you can store any tortillas you don't use in the freezer for up to 3 months.

BELLY BUDDIES:
Maple syrup, lime, olive oil, banana

3 tablespoons pure maple syrup

1 tablespoon fresh lime juice

2 teaspoons extra-virgin olive oil

½ teaspoon ground cinnamon

4 (6-inch) corn tortillas

2 small bananas (5 ounces each), thinly sliced

1. Preheat the oven to 375°F.

2. In a small bowl, stir together the maple syrup, lime juice, oil, and cinnamon.

3. Place the tortillas on a large baking sheet and brush them with half of the maple mixture. Top with the sliced bananas. Brush the banana slices with the remaining maple mixture.

4. Bake for 12 minutes, or until the tortillas are lightly crisped and the bananas are piping hot.

Per tart: 181 calories • 2g protein • 3g fat (0.5g saturated) • 3.5g fiber • 39g carbohydrate • 6mg sodium • 40mg magnesium

Cooking for One: Combine 2¼ teaspoons maple syrup, ¾ teaspoon lime juice, ½ teaspoon olive oil, and a pinch of cinnamon. Brush 1 corn tortilla with half of the mixture, top with ¼ banana and the remaining maple mixture, and bake as directed.

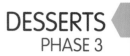

Mochachino Cupcakes

Hands-On Time: 20 minutes | **Total Time:** 40 minutes plus cooling time | **Makes:** 12 cupcakes

These can be wrapped individually and frozen for up to 3 months before icing. Unwrap and thaw at room temperature, then spread the chocolate over the top. Because these are a little more carb-dense than most of the foods on the 21-Day Tummy plan, be sure to stick with Phase 1 recipes and other naturally carb-light foods for the rest of your meal. In addition, cocoa powder is relatively high in FODMAPs but the small amount used in this recipe shouldn't bother your tummy.

1 cup brown rice flour

½ cup packed light brown sugar

¼ cup unsweetened cocoa powder

1 tablespoon espresso powder

1 teaspoon baking powder

¼ teaspoon baking soda

¼ teaspoon salt

⅓ cup unsweetened rice milk

¼ cup extra-virgin olive oil

2 large eggs

1½ teaspoons vanilla extract

1½ ounces semisweet chocolate, coarsely chopped

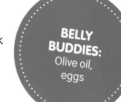

BELLY BUDDIES: Olive oil, eggs

1. Preheat the oven to 350°F. Line 12 cups of a muffin tin with paper liners.

2. In a large bowl, whisk together the flour, brown sugar, cocoa powder, espresso powder, baking powder, baking soda, and salt.

3. In a separate bowl, whisk together the rice milk, oil, eggs, and vanilla. Stir the egg mixture into the flour mixture. Divide the batter among the muffin cups.

4. Bake for 17 minutes, or until the tops of the cupcakes spring back when lightly touched and a toothpick inserted in the center of a cupcake comes out clean.

5. In a small bowl set over (but not in) a pan of simmering water, melt the chocolate. Spread the chocolate over the cooled cupcakes.

Per cupcake: 161 calories • 3g protein • 7g fat (1.5g saturated) • 1.5g fiber • 23g carbohydrate • 139mg sodium • 3mg magnesium

If you have gluten issues: Choose a gluten-free brand of baking powder.

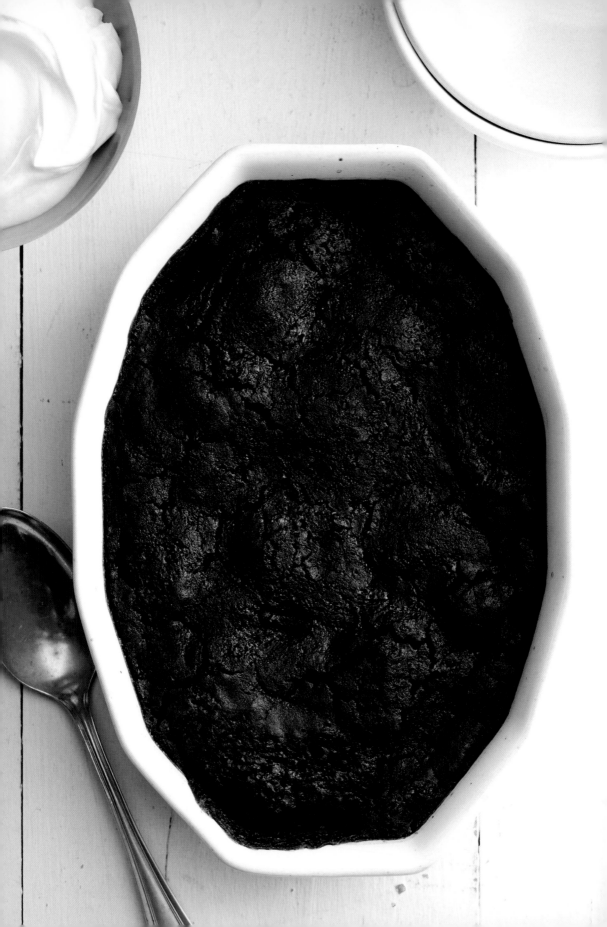

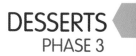

Espresso Pudding Cake

Hands-On Time: 10 minutes | **Total Time:** 30 minutes | **Makes:** 8 servings

This is a very moist cake with streaks of creamy pudding running through it. It's not a cake that you can cut into slices; it's more of a dessert that you scoop into a bowl. The cake actually freezes well, so scoop the leftover cake (in equal portions, one-eighth of the cake) into freezer containers. Reheat in the microwave in 20-second increments until warm.

¼ cup packed turbinado sugar or light brown sugar

2 tablespoons unsweetened cocoa powder

1½ teaspoons instant espresso powder

A pinch plus ⅛ teaspoon salt

¾ cup brown rice flour

1½ teaspoons baking powder

¼ teaspoon ground cinnamon

⅓ cup lactose-free 1% milk

3 tablespoons extra-light olive oil

½ teaspoon vanilla extract

⅓ cup plus 2 tablespoons pure maple syrup

1 cup very hot water

½ cup nonfat plain Greek yogurt

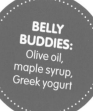

BELLY BUDDIES: Olive oil, maple syrup, Greek yogurt

1. Preheat the oven to 350°F. In a small bowl, stir together the sugar, 1 tablespoon of the cocoa powder, ½ teaspoon of the espresso powder, and a pinch of salt. Set aside.

2. In a medium bowl, combine the flour, baking powder, cinnamon, and the remaining 1 tablespoon cocoa, 1 teaspoon espresso, and ⅛ teaspoon salt.

3. In a 1-cup measure, combine the milk, oil, vanilla, and ⅓ cup of the maple syrup. Stir into the flour mixture until well combined.

4. Scrape the batter into an ungreased 8 x 8-inch baking pan and spread it evenly.

5. Sprinkle the reserved sugar mixture over the batter. Pour the hot water on top and bake for 18 to 20 minutes, or until the top is set and the mixture is bubbling.

6. Meanwhile, in a small bowl, stir together the yogurt and the remaining 2 tablespoons maple syrup.

7. Serve the pudding cake warm or at room temperature, with a dollop of sweetened yogurt on the side.

Per serving: 188 calories • 3g protein • 5.5g fat (1g saturated) • 1g fiber • 33g carbohydrate • 229mg sodium • 6mg magnesium

If you have gluten issues: Choose gluten-free brands of Greek yogurt and baking powder.

Appendix A:
Your Belly Bully Tests

Give yourself a big pat on the back! Cheers to you for prioritizing your health and making the necessary changes in your diet to feel your very best.

In the 21-Day Tummy plan, we took out all of the potentially offending FODMAPs from the diet to ensure that nothing could disturb your belly. But because many FODMAP-containing foods are innately healthy, we don't want you to restrict any of them unnecessarily. So now it's time to identify which FODMAPs are your personal Belly Bullies.

Note that carb-dense foods and pro-inflammatory fats affect everyone the same way, so you don't need to test them. Just keep your consumption to a minimum. The Belly Bully Tests we're presenting here will determine your sensitivity to specific FODMAPs. Remember that each of us has our own personal tolerance to FODMAPs. For instance, I discovered that I can tolerate a little bit of lactose in Greek yogurt and hard cheeses, but foods with excess fructose are a surefire path to bloating and cramping. No fun.

> Because many FODMAP-containing foods are innately healthy, we don't want you to restrict any of them unnecessarily.

Once you've completed the tests, if you still have weight to lose, repeat Phases 2 and 3 of the 21-Day Tummy meal plan, occasionally adding in the Belly Bullies you've just discovered are safe for you. Continue doing that until you've reached your goal weight. Likewise, if you are still experiencing digestive symptoms, cycle through Phases 2 and 3 until you are symptom free.

After you've reached your weight loss and health goals and figured out your personal Belly Bullies, I suggest that you continue to follow Phase 3 of the diet, with the belly-friendly balanced plate you already know how to put together. If digestive symptoms start to flare up again or the pounds start to creep up, simply start the 21-Day Tummy plan over again from Phase 1 to calm and flatten your belly. (So that your body doesn't go into starvation mode, though, do this no more than four times per year.)

Guidelines for the Belly Bully Tests

Here's what you do to identify your personal Belly Bullies:

- Take the tests one at a time. Return to 21-Day Tummy clean eating after you've "passed" each.

- As you take each test, continue to follow the 21-Day Tummy meal plan (but remember that you can pick and choose your favorite meals from any phase). This will ensure you have limited intake of other potential offenders in your diet so it's clear what foods really bother you.

- Challenge the foods in the order provided.

- Consume the amount suggested in each Belly Bully test once per day for 2 to 3 days in a row (unless otherwise noted).

- Stop eating a food if you develop symptoms. Don't start your next test until you are symptom free for 2 to 3 days.

- Track your tests with a food log, whether digital or on paper, recording how much of each test food you ate and when, and whether you develop any sumptoms.

- Because your tolerance to different FODMAPs may change over time—due to changes in your gut bacteria, your stress level, your overall health, and other factors—if you fail a test now, repeat the test again in a few months.

Test Doses for the Belly Bully Test

Here are the Belly Bullies you will be challenging over the next several weeks. Simply add the food described to your daily menu as you see fit.

TEST #1: Lactose

Drink 1 cup milk or eat 1 cup regular (not Greek) yogurt.

If your symptoms flare up after this challenge, avoid lactose-rich dairy products such as milk, yogurt, ice cream, custard, ricotta, and cottage cheese. Switch to lactose-free dairy versions of these foods. Most people digest hard cheeses well since they have less lactose. Greek yogurt is lower in lactose than regular yogurt, but if you're especially sensitive to lactose and you find that even the Greek yogurt gives you tummy trouble, substitute a lactose-free yogurt such as the Green Valley Organics brand.

You could also try lactase enzyme supplements. These enzymes can be purchased at your local drug store and will help your body break lactose down into its digestible sugars, glucose and galactose.

TEST #2: Fructose

Eat ½ a mango or 1–2 teaspoons honey.

If you experience GI symptoms after this challenge, you will want to limit foods or beverages that contain more fructose than glucose. Examples of foods with a high fructose-to-glucose ratio include: apples, pears, mangoes, asparagus, sugar snap peas, honey, agave nectar, and any food containing high-fructose corn syrup.

TEST #3: Sorbitol (a type of polyol)

Eat 2 dried apricots or 1 nectarine.

If you fail this challenge, limit apples, pears, and stone fruits such as peaches, plums, and apricots. Also, avoid gum and mints made with sorbitol.

TEST #4: Mannitol (a type of polyol)

Eat ½ cup mushrooms or ⅓ cup cauliflower.

If you fail this challenge, avoid mushrooms and cauliflower as well as mints and sugar-free gum made with mannitol.

TEST #5: Wheat (a source of fructans)

Eat 2 slices bread or 1 cup cooked pasta (consumed two to three times over the course of 1 week).

If wheat proves to be your downfall, try gluten-free breads, gluten-free pasta, and gluten-free cereals, since they won't contain wheat. (Note that all types of breads and pastas, whether whole grain or white, have fructans.)

TEST #6: Garlic (a source of fructans)

Eat 1 garlic clove (consumed two to three times over the course of 1 week).

If you find garlic doesn't suit you, replace it with the Roasted Garlic Oil recipe (page 211). Commercial soups and dressings often have garlic, so limit or avoid those as well.

TEST #7: Onion (a source of fructans)

Eat 1 tablespoon chopped onion (consumed two to three times over the course of 1 week).

If onions are your problem, replace them with the green part of scallions or perhaps some chives. Avoid commercially made salad dressings and soups, which are rich in onions.

TEST #8: GOS

Eat ½ cup kidney beans, soybeans (edamame), or black beans.

If beans bring on the gas, then simply minimize your bean intake. Canned lentils and chickpeas have lower amounts of GOS compared to other beans, so perhaps try small amounts such as ¼ cup. Or try Beano, a digestive enzyme supplement that may help your body digest GOS more efficiently.

Appendix B:
Belly Bullies

If you stick with the meal-planning guidelines in Chapter 3, I guarantee your belly will feel leaner and cleaner right away. But if you continue to experience digestive symptoms after following the 21-Day Tummy diet for several weeks, you may want to double-check that you haven't inadvertently introduced a Belly Bully. Here's a list of foods to avoid on the plan:

CARB-DENSE FOODS

Bagels

Bread (including whole grain breads)

Cookies

Crackers (including whole wheat crackers and rye crispbreads)

Muffins

Pasta (especially if made with white flour)

Pretzels

Refined cereals (such as cornflakes and puffed rice)

Refined grains (such as white flour and white rice)

Rice cakes (made with white rice)

PRO-INFLAMMATORY FATS

Trans Fats

Fast foods

Packaged foods

Omega-6 Fats

Corn oil

Grapeseed oil

Safflower oil

Soybean oil

Sunflower oil

Saturated Fats

Candy

Fatty cuts of beef

Full-fat dairy products (such as whole milk, butter, and cheese)

Pizza

Processed meat (such as bacon, bologna, hot dogs, pepperoni, salami, and sausages)

HIGH-LACTOSE FOODS

Dairy-based desserts
Cheesecake
Crème brûlée
Flan
Ice cream
Pudding
Tiramisu

Milk (includes whole, low-fat, and skim)
Goat's milk
Evaporated milk
Sheep's milk
Sweetened condensed milk
Milk powder or milk solids

Yogurt
Regular (non-Greek) yogurt

Soft cheeses
Cottage cheese
Crème fraîche
Mascarpone
Ricotta

HIGH-FRUCTOSE FOODS

Fruits
Apples
Cherries
Mangoes
Pears
Watermelon

Vegetables
Artichokes
Asparagus
Fava beans
Sugar snap peas
Sun-dried tomato or tomato paste (if more than 1 tablespoon)

Sweeteners
Agave nectar
Fruit juice concentrate
High-fructose corn syrup
Honey

HIGH-FRUCTAN FOODS

Fruits
Dates
Figs, dried
Grapefruit
Nectarines
Persimmons
Prunes
Raisins
Watermelon
White peaches

Nuts
Cashews
Pistachios

Grains
Barley
Rye
Wheat

Vegetables
Artichokes
Garlic
Leeks (white part)
Onions
Scallions (white part)
Shallots

Legumes
Black beans
Black-eyed peas
Kidney beans
Lima beans
Soybeans

Additives
Inulin (also called chicory root extract)
FOS (fructo-oligosaccharides)

HIGH-GOS (GALACTO-OLIGOSACCHARIDES) FOODS

Beans

Adzuki beans
Black beans
Butter beans
Cannellini beans
Fava beans
Great northern beans

Kidney beans
Lima beans
Mung beans (but bean sprouts are okay)
Navy beans
Pinto beans

Soybeans (but tofu and tempeh are okay)
Split peas

Nuts

Cashews
Pistachios

HIGH-POLYOL FOODS

Fruits

Apples
Apricots
Blackberries
Cherries
Nectarines
Peaches
Pears
Plums
Prunes
Watermelon

Vegetables

Cauliflower
Mushrooms
Snow peas

Sugar-Free Foods

Candy
Gums
Mints

Artificial Sweeteners/Additives

Isomalt
Maltitol
Mannitol
Polydextrose
Sorbitol
Xylitol

NOTES

Chapter 1

1. Harvard School of Public Health, "The Obesity Prevention Source: Obesity Trends," accessed September 10, 2013, www.hsph.harvard.edu/obesity-prevention-source/obesity-trends/.

2. Centers for Disease Control and Prevention, "Overweight and Obesity: Adult Obesity Facts," last modified August 16, 2013, www.cdc.gov/obesity/data/adult.html.

3. "FastStats: Obesity and Overweight," Centers for Disease Control and Prevention, last modified May 30, 2013, www.cdc.gov/nchs/fastats/overwt.htm.

4. B. C. Jacobson et al., "Body-Mass Index and Symptoms of Gastroesophageal Reflux in Women," *New England Journal of Medicine* 354 (2006): 2340–48.

5. E. Ness-Jensen et al., "Changes in Prevalence, Incidence and Spontaneous Loss of Gastro-oesophageal Reflux Symptoms: A Prospective Population-Based Cohort Study, the HUNT Study," Gut 61, no. 10 (October 2011): 1390–97.

6. National Institutes of Health, *Opportunities and Challenges in Digestive Diseases Research: Recommendations of the National Commission on Digestive Diseases*, NIH Publication 08–6514 (2009), www2.niddk.nih.gov/NR/rdonlyres/722FC3D9-B5EC-47AE-8BF5-6DBB8900EAB3/0/NCDD_04272009_ResearchPlan_CompleteResearchPlan.pdf.

7. R. S. Sandler et al., "Abdominal Pain, Bloating, and Diarrhea in the United States: Prevalence and Impact," *Digestive Diseases and Sciences* 45, no. 6 (June 2000): 1166–71.

8. J. K. DiBaise et al., "Gut Microbiota and Its Possible Relationship with Obesity," Mayo Clinic Proceedings 83, no. 4 (April 2008): 460–69.

9. F. Backhed et al., "The Gut Microbiota as an Environmental Factor That Regulates Fat Storage," *Proceedings of the National Academy of Sciences* 101, no. 44 (November 2007): 15718–23.

10. A. Liou et al., "Conserved Shifts in the Gut Microbiota Due to Gastric Bypass Reduces Host Weight and Adiposity," *Science Translational Medicine* 5, no. 178 (March 2013): 178ra41.

11. L. Rigsbee et al., "Quantitative Profiling of Gut Microbiota of Children with Diarrhea Predominant Irritable Bowel Syndrome," *American Journal of Gastroenterology* 107, no. 11 (November 2012): 1740–51.

12. L. Yang et al., "Inflammation and Intestinal Metaplasia of the Distal Esophagus Are Associated with Alterations in the Microbiome," *Gastroenterology* 137, no. 2 (August 2009): 588–97.

13. P. Marteau, "Bacterial Flora in Inflammatory Bowel Disease," supplement, *Digestive Diseases* 27 (2009): S99–103.

14. G. Engstrom et al., "Inflammation-Sensitive Plasma Proteins Are Associated with Future Weight Gain," *Diabetes* 52, no. 8 (August 2003): 2097–2101.

15. D. Tuo et al., "Class II Major Histocompatibility Complex Plays an Essential Role in Obesity-Induced Adipose Inflammation," *Cell Metabolism* 17, no. 3 (March 2013): 411–22.

16. A. K. Gupta et al., "Cardiovascular Risk Escalation with Caloric Excess: A Prospective Demonstration of the Mechanics in Healthy Adults," *Cardiovascular Diabetology* 12, no. 23 (January 2013), www.cardiab.com/content/pdf/1475-2840-12-23.pdf.

17. L. K. Vigsnaes et al., "Gram-Negative Bacteria Account for Main Differences Between Faecal Microbiota from Patients with Ulcerative Colitis and Healthy Controls," *Beneficial Microbes* 3, no. 4 (December 2012): 287–97, www.ncbi.nlm.nih.gov/pubmed/22968374.

18. S. Lindeberg and B. Lundh, "Apparent Absence of Stroke and Ischaemic Heart Disease in a Traditional Melanesian Island: A Clinical Study in Kitava," *Journal of Internal Medicine* 233, no. 3 (March 1993): 269–75.

19. S. Lindeberg et al., "Low Serum Insulin in Traditional Pacific Islanders—The Kitava Study," *Metabolism* 48, no. 10 (1999): 1216–19.

20. S. Lindeberg et al., "Large Differences in Serum Leptin Levels Between Nonwesternized and Westernized Populations: The Kitava Study," *Journal of Internal Medicine* 249, no. 6 (2001): 553–58.

21. I. Spreadbury, "Comparison with Ancestral Diets Suggests Dense Acellular Carbohydrates Promote an Inflammatory Microbiota, and May Be the Primary Dietary Cause of Leptin Resistance and Obesity," *Diabetes, Metabolic Syndrome and Obesity: Targets and Therapy* 5 (July 2012): 175–89.

22. E. Lopez-Garcia et al., "Consumption of Trans Fatty Acids Is Related to Plasma Biomarkers of Inflammation and Endothelial Dysfunction," *Journal of Nutrition* 135, no. 3 (March 2005): 562–66.

23. D. Estadella et al., "Lipotoxicity: Effects of Dietary Saturated and Transfatty Acids," *Mediators of Inflammation* 2013 (January 2013), www.hindawi.com/journals/mi/2013/137579/.

24. J. K. Kiecolt-Glaser et al., "Depressive Symptoms, Omega-6:Omega-3 Fatty Acids, and Inflammation in Older Adults," *Psychosomatic Medicine* 69, no. 3 (April 2007): 217–24.

25. D. E. King et al., "Dietary Magnesium and C-reactive Protein Levels," *Journal of the American College of Nutrition* 24, no. 3 (June 2005): 166–71.

26. Health Canada, "Do Canadian Adults Meet Their Nutrient Requirements Through Food Intake Alone?" accessed September 19, 2013, www.hc-sc.gc.ca/fn-an/alt_formats/pdf/surveill/nutrition/commun/art-nutr-adult-eng.pdf.

27. S. Johnson, "The Multifaceted and Widespread Pathology of Magnesium Deficiency," *Medical Hypotheses* 56, no. 2 (February 2001): 163–70.

28. Y. Rayssiguier et al., "High Fructose Consumption Combined with Low Dietary Magnesium May Increase the Incidence of the Metabolic Syndrome by Inducing Inflammation," *Magnesium Research* 19, no. 4 (December 2006): 237–43.

29. P. D. Higgins and J. F. Johanson, "Epidemiology of Constipation in North America: A Systematic Review," *American Journal of Gastroenterology* 99, no. 4 (April 2004): 750–59.

30. National Institutes of Health, "Heartburn, Gastroesophageal Reflux (GER), and Gastroesophageal Reflux Disease (GERD)," National Digestive Diseases Information Clearinghouse Publication No. 07-0882 (May 2007).

31. E. Ness-Jensen et al., "Changes in Prevalence, Incidence and Spontaneous Loss of Gastro-oesophageal Reflux Symptoms," 1390–97.

32. WebMD, "Digestive Disorders Health Center: The Basics of Constipation," accessed June 24, 2013, www.webmd.com/digestive-disorders/digestive-diseases-constipation.

33. U. C. Ghoshal et al., "Slow Transit Constipation Associated with Excess Methane Production and Its Improvement Following Rifaximin Therapy: A Case Report," *Journal of Neurogastroenterology and Motility* 17, no. 2 (April 2011): 185–88.

34. R. J. Basseri et al., "Intestinal Methane Production in Obese Individuals Is Associated with a Higher Body Mass Index," *Gastroenterology and Hepatology* 8, no. 1 (January 2012): 22–28.

35. J. S. Barrett et al., "Dietary Poorly Absorbed, Short-Chain Carbohydrates Increase Delivery of Water and Fermentable Substrates to the Proximal Colon," *Alimentary Pharmacology Therapeutics* 31, no. 8 (April 2010): 874–82.

36. Mayo Clinic, "Irritable Bowel Syndrome," accessed June 24, 2013, www.mayoclinic.com/health/irritable-bowel-syndrome/DS00106.

37. C. Zacker et al., "Absenteeism Among Employees with Irritable Bowel Syndrome," *Managed Care Interface* 17, no. 5 (May 2004): 28–32.

38. H. M. Staudacher et al., "Comparison of Symptom Response Following Advice for a Diet Low in Fermentable Carbohydrates (FODMAPs) Versus Standard Dietary Advice in Patients with Irritable Bowel Syndrome," *Journal of Human Nutrition and Dietetics* 24, no. 5 (October 2011): 487–95.

39. A. Rubio-Tapio et al., "Increased Prevalence of and Mortality in Undiagnosed Celiac Disease," *Gastroenterology* 137, no. 1 (July 2009): 88–93.

40. University of Maryland Medical Center, "School of Medicine Researchers Identify Key Pathogenic Differences Between Celiac Disease and Gluten Sensitivity," news release, March 10, 2011, www.umm.edu/news/releases/gluten-sensitivity-celiac-disease.htm#ixzz2U1XCd3cP.

Chapter 2

1. J. Jiang et al., "Indole-3-Carbinol Inhibits LPS-Induced Inflammatory Response by Blocking TRIF-Dependent Signaling Pathway in Macrophages," *Food and Chemical Toxicology* 57 (July 2013): 256–61.

2. P. J. Moughan, S. M. Rutherfurd, and P. Balan, "Kiwifruit, Mucins, and the Gut Barrier," *Advances in Food and Nutrition Research* 68 (2013): 169–85.

3. L. Kaur and M. Boland, "Influence of Kiwifruit on Protein Digestion," *Advances in Food and Nutrition Research* 68 (2013): 149–67.

4. M. Kristensen and S. Bügel, "A Diet Rich in Oat Bran Improves Blood Lipids and Hemostatic Factors, and Reduces Apparent Energy Digestibility in Young Healthy Volunteers," *European Journal of Clinical Nutrition* 65, no. 9 (September 2011): 1053–58.

5. M. P. St-Onge et al., "Medium-Chain Triglycerides Increase Energy Expenditure and Decrease Adiposity in Overweight Men," *Obesity Research* 11, no. 3 (March 2003): 395–402.

6. K. L. Wu et al., "Effects of Ginger on Gastric Emptying and Motility in Healthy Humans," *European Journal of Gastroenterology and Hepatology* 20, no. 5 (May 2008): 436–40.

7. G. Ramadan, M. A. Al-Kahtani, and W. M. El-Sayed, "Anti-inflammatory and Anti-oxidant Properties of Curcuma longa (Turmeric) Versus Zingiber officinale (Ginger) Rhizomes in Rat Adjuvant-Induced Arthritis," *Inflammation* 34, no. 4 (August 2011): 291–301.

8. H. Hanai and K. Sugimoto, "Curcumin Has Bright Prospects for the Treatment of Inflammatory Bowel Disease," *Current Pharmaceutical Design* 15, no. 18 (2009): 2087–94.

9. L. Li and N. P. Seeram, "Further Investigation into Maple Syrup Yields 3 New Lignans, a New Phenylpropanoid, and 26 Other Phytochemicals," *Journal of Agricultural and Food Chemistry* 59, no. 14 (July 2011): 7708–16.

Chapter 3

1. B. Sears and C. Ricordi, "Anti-Inflammatory Nutrition as a Pharmacological Approach to Treat Obesity," *Journal of Obesity* 2011 (2011), www.hindawi.com/journals/jobes/2011/431985/.

Recipe Index

PHASE 1

Index

Conversion Charts

ABBREVIATIONS

C	Celsius
cm	centimeter
F	Fahrenheit
fl oz	fluid ounce
ft	foot
g	gram
gal	gallon
in.	inch
kg	kilogram
L	liter
lb	pound
m	meter
mL	milliliter
mm	millimeter
oz	ounce
qt	quart
tbsp	tablespoon
tsp	teaspoon

TEASPOONS

⅛ tsp	0.5 mL
¼ tsp	1 mL
½ tsp	2 mL
¾ tsp	4 mL
1 tsp	5 mL
1½ tsp	7 mL
2 tsp	10 mL

TABLESPOONS

1 tbsp	15 mL
1½ tbsp	20 mL
2 tbsp	30 mL
3 tbsp	45 mL
4 tbsp	60 mL
5 tbsp	75 mL
6 tbsp	90 mL
8 tbsp	125 mL

WEIGHTS

1 oz	30 g
2 oz	60 g
3 oz	90 g
4 oz	125 g
5 oz	150 g
6 oz	175 g
8 oz	250 g
10 oz	300 g
12 oz	375 g
16 oz	500 g
32 oz	1 kg
¼ lb	125 g
½ lb	250 g
⅔ lb	300 g
¾ lb	375 g
1 lb	500 g
2 lb	1 kg
3 lb	1.5 kg

LENGTHS

¼ in.	5 mm
½ in.	1 cm
1 in.	2.5 cm
2 in.	5 cm
6 in.	15 cm
1 ft	30 cm

VOLUME

1 fl oz	30 mL
2 fl oz	50 mL
5 fl oz	150 mL
10 fl oz	300 mL
1 pint	500 mL
1 qt	1 L
1 gal	4 L
¼ cup	60 mL
⅓ cup	75 mL
½ cup	125 mL
⅔ cup	150 mL
¾ cup	175 mL
1 cup	250 mL
1¼ cups	300 mL
1½ cups	375 mL
2 cups	500 mL
4 cups	1 L
6 cups	1.5 L

OVEN TEMPERATURES

°F	°C
175°F	80°C
200°F	95°C
225°F	110°C
250°F	120°C
275°F	140°C
300°F	150°C
325°F	160°C
350°F	180°C
375°F	190°C
400°F	200°C
425°F	220°C
450°F	230°C
475°F	240°C
500°F	260°C

BAKING PANS

8 x 8 in.	20 x 20 cm
9 x 9 in.	22 x 22 cm
9 x 13 in.	22 x 33 cm
10 x 15 in.	25 x 38 cm
11 x 17 in.	28 x 43 cm
8 x 2 in. (round)	20 x 5 cm
9 x 2 in. (round)	22 x 5 cm
10 x 4½ in. (tube)	25 x 11 cm
8 x 4 x 3 in. (loaf)	20 x 10 x 7.5 cm
9 x 5 x 3 in. (loaf)	22 x 12.5 x 7.5 cm

CASSEROLE DISHES

Recipe calls for	Substitute
1 qt (4 cups)	900 mL
1½ qt (6 cups)	1.35 L
2–2½ qt (8–10 cups)	2.25 L
3 qt (12 cups)	2.7 L
4–5 qt (16–20 cups)	4.5 L